# PRAISE FOR
## THIS ISN'T WHAT I E...

"Practical, purposeful, and passionate, this new edition of *This Isn't What I Expected* will continue to be an invaluable resource for postpartum moms, their families, and their friends. Karen Kleiman, MSW, and Valerie Raskin, MD, share their wealth of clinical experience with a clear and engaging style that makes this now classic self-help book the perfect contemporary guide to finding the help you need now."
   —Shari I. Lusskin, MD, Adjunct Associate Professor of Psychiatry, Obstetrics, Gynecology, and Reproductive Sciences, The Icahn School of Medicine at Mount Sinai

"What you can expect from this classic book on postpartum mood and anxiety disorders is the most current information delivered in a sensitive and understandable format. Kleiman and Raskin help you identify and navigate the complexities of postpartum depression and anxiety beyond just recognizing symptoms. With insight, empathy, and vast experience in the field of maternal mental health they offer explanations and practical strategies that lead you to recovery and protect against relapse. *This Isn't What I Expected* belongs on the bookshelf of every new mom, dad, and the care providers who treat them"
   —Diana Lynn Barnes, PsyD, The Center for Postpartum Health, Co-author of *The Journey to Parenthood: Myths, Reality and What Really Matters.*

"*This Isn't What I Expected: Overcoming Postpartum Depression* was instrumental in helping me recover from severe postpartum depression. The book not only helped me understand what was happening to me during the most puzzling and terrifying time in my life, but empowered me with tools to cope through the utter despair."

—Sandra Poulin, author of *The Mother-To-Mother Postpartum Depression Support Book: Real Stories from Women Who Lived Through It and Recovered*

"In this second edition of *This Isn't What I Expected*, the authors describe the knowledge gained over the past 15–20 years in the growing field of perinatal psychiatry. The authors bring together the facts about postpartum mood disorders in a concise and readable fashion. They address a variety of topics from treatment to prevention and offer essential information such as identification of symptoms, resources for treatment and support, and behavioral techniques to manage symptoms. This new volume is a significant contribution to our growing field of perinatal psychiatry, and a gift to the mothers, infants and families we serve."

—Margaret Spinelli, MD, Associate Professor of Clinical Psychiatry, Columbia University College of Physicians and Surgeons; Director, Maternal Mental Health Program

*This Isn't*
*What I Expected*

*l Edition*

# This Isn't
# What I Expected

..⦂❩ *Overcoming Postpartum Depression* ❨⦂..

**Karen Kleiman, MSW, LCSW
and Valerie Davis Raskin, MD**

Da Capo

**LIFE
LONG**

A Member of the Perseus Books Group

Designed by Linda Mark
Set in12 point Joanna MT Std by the Perseus Books Group

Library of Congress Cataloging-in-Publication Data

Kleiman, Karen R.
  This isn't what I expected: overcoming postpartum depression / Karen R.
Kleiman, MSW, LCSW, and Valerie Davis Raskin, MD.—Second edition.
    pages cm
  Includes bibliographical references and index.
  ISBN 978-0-7382-1693-5 (pbk.)—ISBN 978-0-7382-1694-2 (e-book)
  1.Postpartum depression.  I. Raskin, Valerie D. II. Title.
RG852.K56 2013
618.7'6—dc23

                                                    2013028232

First Da Capo Press edition 2013
Published by Da Capo Press
A Member of the Perseus Books Group
www.dacapopress.com

Note: The information in this book is true and complete to the best of our
knowledge. This book is intended only as an informative guide for those
wishing to know more about health issues. In no way is this book intended
to replace, countermand, or conflict with the advice given to you by your
own physician. The ultimate decision concerning care should be made between
you and your doctor. We strongly recommend you follow his or her advice.
Information in this book is general and is offered with no guarantees on the
part of the authors or Da Capo Press. The authors and publisher disclaim all
liability in connection with the use of this book. The names and identifying
details of people associated with events described in this book have been
changed. Any similarity to actual persons is coincidental.

Da Capo Press books are available at special discounts for bulk purchases in
the United States by corporations, institutions, and other organizations. For
more information, please contact the Special Markets Department at the
Perseus Books Group, 2300 Chestnut Street, Suite 200, Philadelphia, PA, 19103,
or call (800) 810-4145, ext. 5000, or e-mail special.markets@perseusbooks.com.

10 9 8 7 6 5 4 3 2 1

*For our mothers, Miriam and Mary.*

# CONTENTS

# INTRODUCTION

*W*HEN WE WROTE THE FIRST comprehensive guide for postpartum depression, *This Isn't What I Expected*, almost two decades ago, we surely hoped that things would be different by now: mothers wouldn't feel so much pressure to be perfect, the link between hormones and postpartum depression would be well understood, new medications would work quickly and without side effects, and society would support young families, as is done in some parts of the world, with generous parental leaves and flexible work schedules. Maternal love wouldn't be evaluated by whether a woman works in the home full time, not at all, or something in between. Women with postpartum depression and anxiety wouldn't be judged as either trying too hard or not trying hard enough. Every obstetrician would know that postpartum emotional disorders are the most frequent medical complication of childbirth, and therefore all new parents would be screened and educated about this disorder.

We were certain that the stigma and shame of postpartum depression (PPD) and anxiety would lessen. We imagined that by the time our daughters become mothers, everyone would laugh at the quaint notion that postpartum depression was any less "real" than anemia or an infected milk duct.

Some things *are* better these days. Thanks to prominent celebrity moms such as Brooke Shields, Gwyneth Paltrow, and Marie Osmond, who bravely discussed their own struggles with PPD, most of us now recognize that this illness truly can happen to anyone. There are better resources and treatment options than ever before. There are some newer medications, none perfect, and we know more about breastfeeding and medication safety than we used to.

Public awareness has definitely improved. As clinicians, researchers, and advocates for women's healthcare, we both are thrilled to have witnessed and been a part of these important advancements. Even so, it saddens us that our communities and larger society haven't made all the progress women who are having difficulty after childbirth deserve. It remains frustrating that postpartum depression is still perceived as a personal weakness; that a suicidal mom may still be afraid to disclose how she is feeling; and that some doctors still mistake postpartum suffering for normal postpartum adjustment.

In updating the book, we were not surprised to find outdated references to portable cassette players and $3.00-an-hour babysitters. What did surprise us, though, was how relevant the majority of the book's messages and recommendations remain to this day. For some thirty years we have been treating women with postpartum depression and anxiety. And though we have newer medications with fewer side effects, welcomed legislation, greater public awareness, and more research to validate treatment options, one truth has proven to be constant: women with PPD continue to wait apprehensively in the dark corners of their lives, fearful of judgment, stigma, ridicule, and misdiagnosis. They wait, hoping this will go away by itself, hoping they will not go completely mad, hoping they do not have to let anyone know how they are really feeling.

Because of the increase in public awareness, more women have heard of PPD, but they continue to believe "that couldn't happen to me." No one expects to get depressed after they have a baby. Yet women may be vulnerable to depression after childbirth for many reasons. They may have gone through painful, lengthy infertility treatments, certain that a baby would bring nothing but joy. They may have expected their partners to be like Hollywood dads: doing half the work. They may be very accomplished women who find themselves helpless when it comes to soothing a colicky baby. They may be deeply affected by hard economic times, struggling with their own unemployment, or their partners'. They may be terrified by the ongoing media fascination with the extremely rare mother with postpartum psychosis, afraid that someone will think they are a danger to their beloved children.

And so, again, we present this book to the postpartum woman and her family, to ensure that accurate information is getting into the hands of the families who need it most. It is generally accepted that approximately one in seven postpartum women suffer from a serious mood disorder, referred to clinically as a major depressive disorder (MDD). The statistics are even more striking (one in five postpartum women) when referring to the entire spectrum of postpartum disorders that encompasses postpartum depression, postpartum anxiety, postpartum panic, postpartum obsessive-compulsive disorder (OCD), and postpartum post-traumatic stress disorder (PTSD). We also offer this book to women who are not experiencing full-blown postpartum depression. Another whopping 20–30 percent of new mothers won't ever meet diagnostic criteria for PPD, but they feel terrible and are not sure what is wrong. They may cry at times, may feel overwhelmed on occasion, and may have moments of despair or panic. We call this phenomenon postpartum stress syndrome. When it comes to the anticipated joy of new motherhood, the painful reality is that only one in two women find that motherhood is all that it's cracked up to be. If you take nothing else away from this book, we hope that you come to know that you are not the only one and you are not to blame.

When we initially set out to write this book, we were both young mothers ourselves, dedicated to our work, with the challenges and joys that accompany this time in a woman's life. Since that time, our own cribs have been replaced by empty nests, giving us a new perspective from which we now continue to observe and learn. And sadly, we have come to realize that some things have not changed much. Postpartum women continue to suffer in silence. So much so that "suffering in silence" is paraphrased throughout countless worldwide campaigns to raise PPD awareness. From New Zealand to Durango, from the US National Library of Medicine at the National Institutes of Health to *The Tyra Show*, "suffering in silence" has become a hallmark expression to depict the isolation that is so characteristic of this illness. Women are still not talking about how they are feeling. They are still not sure that they are safe to disclose their scary symptoms. They are still not convinced they won't be judged, or misunderstood, or locked away, or labeled crazy. Similarly, healthcare providers remain locked into unproductive patterns that do little to encourage postpartum women to speak out. Some fail to ask the right questions. Some fail to refer appropriately after screening. Some hand out a prescription for antidepressants without adequate probing or follow-up. Some believe that postpartum depression doesn't exist or is synonymous with baby blues or with psychosis. Others think their patients would feel better if they had more sex or a date night with their partner.

It is still, therefore, up to each individual woman and her family to ensure that she is getting good, accurate information and exposing herself to state-of-the-art treatment or self-help strategies that have been shown to be effective when managing symptoms of depression or anxiety during the postpartum period. Self-help books can be extremely helpful, particularly during the postpartum time frame when women are often encumbered by time and financial constraints, schedules, exhaustion, and so on. Women have told us that our book was a "lifeline" and their "bible" when they were struggling with acute symptoms. One woman said, "This book was the next best thing to having you right there with me at home." For these reasons, we believe in the value of the printed word and aim to reach the large number of postpartum women who need support, information, and hope during this difficult time.

These words from our original preface are still true: "The syndrome of depression and anxiety after childbirth is a common disorder that can strike any mother. . . . We have yet to see a woman suffering from postpartum depression who expected it—we all have grown up expecting that this would be one of the best times of our lives . . . Although postpartum illness affects each individual woman in a unique way, many of the issues precipitated by this crisis are very similar among its sufferers."

There is more information available to the consumer than ever before. With the click of a mouse you now have access to more theories, facts, and opinions on postpartum depression than ever before. You can find sound advice, and you can find false claims, such as the assertion that avoiding chocolate will help PPD. Now, more than ever, you need to trust your sources and be discriminate about the knowledge you seek to help you feel better. Sometimes, there is so much information and so much advice; it's hard to know which way to turn. We want to help you with that. Together, we have over fifty years of experience helping women overcome postpartum depression. We've taught over 1,000 healthcare professionals about caring for women with PPD and their families. We've done the research, and we've read the literature. We've seen women get better, and we are familiar with the techniques and interventions that have helped smooth their way. We hope that this book will help you if you or someone you care about is experiencing PPD. We also hope that this book will help to continue to increase public awareness of PPD, and lessen the shame and isolation that makes this disorder so devastating.

# "I Haven't Been Myself Since My Baby Was Born"

## *Recognizing Postpartum Depression*

*"Will I ever feel like myself again?" asks Michelle. "Why am I so sad and irritable all of the time? Is this how it always is after you have a baby?"*

*"Will my wife ever be like she used to be?" asks Jim. "What is happening to Michelle? Why didn't anyone tell us to expect this?"*

MICHELLE* HAS POSTPARTUM DEPRESSION. She—like many women who have given birth—is experiencing difficulty adjusting to this transition in her life. Michelle and Jim can't believe this is happening to them. They were excited about her pregnancy, which was planned and uneventful, and they were well prepared for the birth. They could foresee no problems, and, in fact, when their Lamaze instructor mentioned baby blues and postpartum depression, both thought to themselves, "that couldn't happen to us."

---

\* The names and identifying information of the women and their families who appear throughout this book have been changed to protect their privacy.

Apart from a mild case of the blues for a few hours during the first week after her daughter was born, Michelle felt great for the first month. But then she started feeling down and couldn't sleep well, even though she was always tired. Since she knew that it was not unusual to feel a little sad and moody after having a baby, Michelle tried to dismiss her moodiness and go through the motions of motherhood as best she could. At first, she didn't tell anyone—not even Jim—how poorly she was feeling. By now she was crying at the littlest thing, sometimes at nothing at all. Frightened and unable to sleep, Michelle was constantly comparing herself to other mothers: They *all* look prettier, skinnier, and better dressed than I do. They *all* instinctively know how to be good mothers. And they *all* appear to be doing everything right, effortlessly. Michelle kept criticizing herself: Why can't I do anything right? Why do I feel so overwhelmed and anxious all the time?

At first, Jim was totally supportive. But then, as Michelle was getting worse, he became less and less understanding. Confused and overwhelmed himself, he's now torn between what he thinks Michelle needs, what their baby needs, and what his boss demands: to buck up and get back to work. None of his friends seem to have gone through anything like this, and he finds himself wondering why Michelle can't just snap out of it, like his mother said she should.

Surprised at how familiar this sounds?

PPD frequently strikes without warning—in women without any past emotional problems, without any history of depression, and without any complications in pregnancy. PPD strikes mothers who are in very satisfying marriages, in difficult marriages, or who are single, lesbian, or cohabitating. It strikes women who had easy pregnancies and deliveries, as well as women who suffered prolonged, complicated labors and caesarean sections. It may occur after the first baby, or after the third or fourth. PPD may strike women who promised themselves, "I'll never be like my mother," or women who said, "If only I can be half as good as my mom was raising me." In short, PPD can strike any woman and almost always comes as a shock, not at all what the new parents expected.

Postpartum depression can be devastating physically and emotionally to the new parents. But others feel its effects as well. Friends and family, eager to help out after the birth, may begin to feel frustrated or baffled when it seems that nothing they do appears to do any good. Their feelings hurt, they begin to drop by less often and to offer less assistance. As the new parents' support systems gradually weaken, PPD takes a turn for the worse.

Even though PPD is very common, only a small fraction of women who experience it ever get the help they need. PPD often "falls through the cracks" in the medical profession. If a woman turns to her obstetrician, she may be told that she is just going through a "period of adjustment," and that "all mothers go through this." Meanwhile, her pediatrician may be focusing on the baby, and probably will not ask her how *she* is feeling. If she goes to a therapist, she may be told that her depression is not related to having a baby, and that recent childbirth is merely a "coincidence." At home, her husband may be too overwhelmed himself to be emotionally available to her, or he may fail to recognize that she is suffering from a real illness. Most days, she is alone: in today's society, extended families are rarely available, and thus a ready-made network including the woman's mother, aunts, sisters, and in-laws is not there to help her cope with her experience. And often, even when there are relatives nearby, they can't relate to her difficulty, because their own postpartum experiences were different.

## Do I Have Postpartum Depression?

The concept of depression is often used in our everyday language to refer to rather trivial bad feelings, such as, "OMG! I was so depressed when they told me there weren't any tickets left!" In contrast to the layman's use, the term *depression* has two precise meanings when used by physicians and mental-health professionals: it refers either to an incessant and intense sad, empty feeling, or to the mood disorder called clinical depression, which is characterized by this feeling for two or more weeks.

Postpartum depression means that, after childbirth, a woman exhibits the emotional and physical symptoms of the syndrome of clinical depression. Before getting to the specific symptoms, it may be helpful to clarify why the term *syndrome* is used. In medicine, a "syndrome" refers to those illnesses for which a specific single cause is not known and that have a very typical pattern of symptoms clustering together. For example, respiratory distress syndrome describes a certain pattern of breathing difficulty that may have many different causes, or even an unknown cause. On the other hand, pneumococcal pneumonia is a very specific disease—not a syndrome—caused by a single known bacteria, with specific diagnostic tests and specific antibiotic treatment.

As will be discussed later in this chapter, PPD is a syndrome that does not have one single cause. The fact that depression and anxiety after childbirth are a syndrome and not a specific disease is a major reason why PPD often goes undetected or is misdiagnosed. It is also often a major source of frustration to those suffering from PPD, who would understandably like to have a specific blood test or something like an X-ray to confirm the diagnosis. For the purposes of this book, we will use the abbreviation PPD to include the entire spectrum of postpartum depression, anxiety, and stress reactions. If we are discussing some aspect unique to one disorder, we will make that clear. Otherwise, we use the term PPD for the range of anxiety and mood disorders that occur after childbirth.

We find that many women suffering from PPD don't realize it. Those who do may put off getting help or deny the problem. To make you a better advocate for yourself, we are including several symptom lists that may help you decide whether you have enough symptoms to suspect the diagnosis of PPD. Our lists are designed to help you assess whether you may be suffering from PPD, so you can then take the steps needed to recover. No list of symptoms will ever replace a careful, individual diagnostic assessment from a professional. Keep in mind that certain physical illnesses (such as a thyroid hormone imbalance and anemia) can also masquerade as PPD. Therefore, you should have a complete physical examination before you and/or your therapist decide that you have PPD.

## POSTPARTUM DEPRESSION SYMPTOM CHECKLIST

The following is a list of ways you might be feeling now. These are statements often made by women suffering from PPD. Look over the list and check any statements that correspond to your own feelings.

_____ 1. I can't shake feeling depressed no matter what I do.

_____ 2. I cry at least once a day.

_____ 3. I feel sad most or all of the time.

_____ 4. I can't concentrate.

_____ 5. I don't enjoy the things that I used to enjoy.

_____ 6. I have no interest in making love at all, even though my doctor says I'm now physically able to resume sexual relations.

_____ 7. I can't sleep, even when my baby sleeps.

_____ 8. I feel like a failure all of the time.

_____ 9. I have no energy; I am tired all the time.

_____ 10. I have no appetite and no enjoyment of food (or, I am having sugar and carbohydrate cravings and compulsively eating all the time).

_____ 11. I can't remember the last time I laughed.

_____ 12. Every little thing gets on my nerves lately. Sometimes, I am even furious at my baby. Often, I am angry with my husband.

_____ 13. I feel that the future is hopeless.

_____ 14. It seems like I will feel this way forever.

_____ 15. There are times when I feel that it would be better to be dead than to feel this way for one more minute.

Although most new mothers will easily relate to one or two of the statements listed above, they also will have periods of good feelings and see that things will improve as this transition period progresses. However, women with PPD usually agree with many or even all of the statements included here and generally feel these symptoms most or all of each and every day. *If you agreed with four or more of these statements, you may be suffering from postpartum depression.* Typically, PPD is only diagnosed when these symptoms have lasted for two or more weeks.

As an example, consider Joanne's story:

For the first five weeks after her baby was born, Joanne felt proud of how well everything was going. Although worn down by night after night of interrupted sleep, she enjoyed her baby and wanted her three-month maternity leave to last forever. But one night, instead of collapsing into sleep the minute the baby went down for the four-hour stretch Joanne and Dave called "night," Joanne couldn't fall asleep for two hours. The next night, even though she was exhausted, she actually tossed and turned for three hours, and had only just fallen asleep when the baby awoke for another bottle. The same thing happened the next two nights.

For the next few days, Joanne worried about not going to sleep at night. Then, she began to worry about other things as well—day and night—and could not be reassured by anyone. She cried at the drop of a hat and became so anxious and sad that she lost all interest in food, in leaving the house—in anything but the absolute necessities of getting through the day. She started writing lists of things to remember, because her once razor-sharp memory was useless. When her husband made the minor complaint that she had forgotten to pick up his shirts at the laundry, Joanne sobbed for two straight hours, in agony at what seemed like a bottomless black pit with no way out.

If Joanne were to look over the preceding list, she would see that she had at least half of the symptoms of postpartum depression. She would check the statements about daily crying (number 2), sad feelings most of the time (number 3), difficulty concentrating (number 4), insomnia (number 7), loss of appetite (number 10), hopelessness (number 13), and feeling that this blackness will go on forever (number 14).

Women who have never suffered from PPD or any other form of depression often ask us: "How can I know if I'm experiencing postpartum depression?" The single best way is to trust your own instincts. If you feel that something is wrong, chances are very good that you are right. You know best whether you have experienced a significant postpartum change in your mood, personality, functioning, or ability to cope. Trust yourself, and don't let others dismiss or minimize your situation. For example, Joanne knew something was terribly wrong, especially because she had felt fine for the first five weeks after childbirth. Fortunately for her, when she made an appointment with her obstetrician to talk over her symptoms, her doctor immediately recognized that Joanne had PPD.

## What Causes Postpartum Depression?

At the present time, we cannot say for certain what causes PPD. Most likely, it is caused by a number of factors that vary from individual to individual. Factors that are believed to contribute to PPD include the following: genetic predisposition (i.e., presence of depression in a blood relative); chronic sleep deprivation and fatigue; colicky, hard-to-care-for babies; dramatic hormonal changes; medical complications in either mother or infant; a predisposition to self-criticism; previous postpartum or other type of clinical depression; absence of support from family or friends; and/or isolation.

Hormones likely play a major role in PPD. We say *likely*, because much too little careful, scientifically sound research has been done in this area. However, we now know that adoption puts a woman at risk for PPD, and approximately 10 percent of fathers get depressed after the birth of their baby, so we have evidence that it is not exclusively caused by hormonal factors, at least not for all women. But the profound nature of postpartum hormone changes is so striking that many specialists, including ourselves, believe that further research will implicate hormones in at least some if not almost all forms of PPD. We suspect that the brain chemistry involved may be like a stone thrown into a pool of water: the cascading ripples move across the entire body of water. Changes in reproductive hormones may make waves in other areas of the brain.

Female reproductive hormones have many significant effects on the brain chemicals (*neurotransmitters*) responsible for communication between brain cells, including how much of the neurotransmitter is present, the length of time it is present between cells, and how the receiving cell is affected by the incoming neurotransmitter. The neurotransmitters serotonin, norepinephrine, dopamine, and acetylcholine are known to be out of balance in serious emotional or psychiatric illnesses. In fact, many studies have documented low levels of the metabolites (the breakdown by-products) of these neurotransmitters in the blood, urine, and cerebrospinal fluid (which bathes the brain) in clinically depressed people. Most mental-health researchers agree that dysregulation of these neurotransmitters is a causative factor in clinical depression. Each of these neurotransmitters is modulated by female reproductive hormones.

During pregnancy, reproductive hormones circulate in the bloodstream at much higher levels than at any other time in a woman's life. The placenta itself is the major source of progesterone and estrogen, which means that these hormones drop precipitously within hours of delivery of the placenta. The effect of this sudden hormone change is similar to, though much more intense than, the premenstrual drop in estrogen and progesterone, which appears to cause depressive symptoms (PMS) in a significant number of women. Many other hormones also drop off over the first few postpartum hours, days, and weeks, including prolactin, cortisol, and human chorionic gonadotropin (HCG). The placenta also stimulates production of endorphins, naturally occurring opioids that promote a general sense of well-being and act as nature's obstetric anesthesia. Endorphin levels fall abruptly after childbirth, as they do during the premenstrual phase of a woman's cycle. One hypothesis linking depressive symptoms of PPD and PMS suggests that the fall in endorphins is responsible.

At least half of clinically depressed people have a detectable abnormality in the neuroendocrine system, called the hypothalamic-pituitary-adrenal axis, that shows up as an abnormality of cortisol (a naturally occurring steroid hormone secreted by the adrenal glands) regulation. Many show another sign of hormonal dysregulation in which their pituitary fails to react to the chemical signal to release a hormone to stimulate the thyroid. The hypothalamic-pituitary-adrenal axis is dramatically affected by childbearing, and it may be that although all women experience these hormonal changes, some are vulnerable to experiencing depression and anxiety as a result. The thyroid gland is very significantly affected by childbearing, and we know that even subclinical cases of low thyroid can cause depression.

The jury is still out on which one—or what combination—of these neurochemical agents initiates PPD. Unfortunately, there are no laboratory tests that can be used to make a clinical diagnosis of PPD at present. Our own clinical experience suggests that it is unlikely that there is a single cause for all sufferers. On one end of the spectrum are women who have what seems to be a "pure" biologic disease. They have very strong biologic symptoms, such as insomnia, weight loss, extreme fatigue, profound difficulty getting out of bed in the morning, inability to function even minimally, and/or hallucinations. For other women, massive stress seems to be the major cause. Still others will feel that events in their past (such as having been abused or neglected) have left them vulnerable to depression during any major life crisis. Some have elements of each.

PPD typically occurs one to three months after childbirth. However, PPD can emerge any time from immediately following the birth of the baby until a year after. Some postpartum specialists expand the range to up to three years after giving birth, emphasizing the stressful role that caring for young children plays. Sometimes, when PPD is identified in the latter part of the first postpartum year, it is discovered that the mother actually had some earlier symptoms that were denied, ignored, or misunderstood. There have been cases in which PPD surfaced many months postpartum without previous symptoms, sometimes but not always around the time of weaning or resumed menses, both events associated with major hormonal changes. In some cases—in retrospect—the first symptoms of PPD may have started during pregnancy, but were either mistaken for physical discomforts of pregnancy or minimized as "just moodiness."

Suffering is suffering, whatever its cause. PPD is a real illness; it is not some sort of punishment for moral weakness, self-indulgence, a wish for a boy when you had a girl, a wish for a girl when you had a boy, nor is it anyone's fault. Recognizing the roots of your own PPD will be important in developing a plan for recovery. Many women have a sense of which factors contribute to their pain, and we encourage you to follow your instincts about what you will need to do to recover.

Understanding that PPD has physiological, psychological, and environmental causative factors may help you validate your own experience and may help others close to you recognize that PPD is a real disease, not something you brought on yourself. As we learn more and more about the chemical imbalances that contribute to PPD, however, it is important not to dismiss the trauma of a woman suffering PPD as "just a biological crisis." No woman is just a disease, or just a chemical imbalance. Some (but not all) women will find that when the acute PPD is gone, they discover significant personality or life-experience issues that appear to have predisposed them to the crisis.

Many women wonder how postpartum depression is either different from or the same as clinical depression (that is, depression that is not linked to childbearing). Sometimes, the symptoms are indeed similar or even identical. However, PPD differs from other forms of clinical depression in specific ways. The first major difference is that PPD occurs in the context of a lifelong expectation of what motherhood will be like, including deep-seated dreams, values, hopes, and beliefs about giving birth. The myth that the postpartum period is unequivocally delightful is very widespread, and the woman who suffers from PPD has to struggle with the disappointments of expectations she may have cultivated for most of her life. The often relentless comments by others—"Aren't you thrilled? Isn't having a baby wonderful? Isn't this as great as life gets?"—may only increase her sense of guilt for having less-than-ecstatic thoughts.

The second difference is that PPD occurs at perhaps the most demanding time of a woman's life. The overwhelming responsibility of caring for an infant, the chronic sleep deprivation, and the stress of physical healing can exacerbate symptoms of depression and make recovery more difficult. In addition, the stakes often seem impossibly high: Will this hurt my baby? Does this mean I shouldn't have more children? Does this mean I have to give up nursing my baby? Does this make me an unfit mother?

## What Else Causes Depression and Anxiety After Childbirth?

Clinical depression is only one of a variety of conditions that may cause depression and anxiety after childbirth. The most common of these is baby blues, but this is usually short-lived and mild. Another condition is postpartum stress syndrome, which is the single most common cause of persistent depression and anxiety after childbirth. Finally, there are two postpartum anxiety syndromes called postpartum panic disorder and postpartum obsessive-compulsive disorder.

## IS BABY BLUES THE SAME THING AS POSTPARTUM DEPRESSION?

Baby blues often happens just after giving birth. Vicky's case is typical:

> Everything went the way Vicky thought it would: labor was awful,
> but it only lasted twelve hours, the epidural went in easily and helped
> her through the worst part, and her son, John, was perfect. She felt
> like she was on a natural "high"—so excited that she couldn't wait to
> go home and never again have to let the nurses or doctors take John
> away, even for a few minutes. She and John were home thirty-six
> hours after his birth, and Vicky was pleased that her mother would
> be flying in from out of town within a few days.
>
> The first night went okay, but by the next afternoon, she started
> feeling overwhelmed. The frequent diaper changes, the sleeplessness,
> the constant phone calls, and the mess of the house were getting to
> her. Vicky found herself nursing John in front of the TV, watching a
> talk show about the plight of former child actors, a topic she'd never
> cared about before. Suddenly, she started sobbing, wondering if John
> could ever end up like the people on the show. She felt ridiculous:
> How could she be worrying about something that she knew wouldn't
> ever happen? Later, a TV advertisement for cellular phone service left
> her in tears, wavering between joy and grief. Watching the vignette,
> in which a teenage boy calls a girl he met at summer camp, led her
> to fantasize about what kind of person John would be and how she
> couldn't wait to meet his first girlfriend. Her next thought was how
> hard it would be to see John grow up—everyone was always telling
> her to "enjoy these days because they are over before you blink."
>
> *Am I nuts?* She wondered. This is a four-day-old baby, for heaven's
> sake! Just then, her girlfriend dropped by with a casserole. Vicky cried
> even harder: I'm so lucky to have such caring friends. But when her
> friend exclaimed, "Aha! Looks like a rip-roaring case of baby blues,"
> Vicky felt that she was laughing at her and snapped, "Thanks for the
> brilliant deduction, Sherlock. Don't you have to be someplace?"

Fortunately, Vicky's mood swings settled down within days, and she knew deep down that her friend was right. She wasn't sure what helped, whether it was having her mother there for support, getting over the excruciatingly painful breast engorgement, finally feeling less sore when she sat down, or if her hormones had simply calmed down, but by the seventh day after giving birth, she felt that someone or something had helped her off the emotional roller coaster she had been on.

*Baby blues* (also called *postpartum blues*) is actually not an illness, and it will resolve on its own. It is often confused with PPD, however, because sadness and crying are so common in both conditions. An estimated 60–80 percent of women who give birth experience a brief, temporary moodiness, sometimes with crying, sadness, irritability, or frustration. This typically begins on the third to fifth postpartum day (usually about the time milk production starts) and usually lasts only a few hours or days. Unlike PPD, in baby blues the sadness and crying come and go, are interspersed with periods of serenity and pleasure, and can usually be shaken off with support, a nap, or by getting out of the house.

Baby blues is brought on by the coincidence of several major rapid changes: hormone decreases, breast engorgement, and the transition from the hospital to home. Some studies have implicated plunging levels of estrogens, progesterone, cortisol, and prolactin, but at least one contradictory study has failed to show any association between each hormone and baby blues. Michael O'Hara, PhD, and his colleagues at the University of Iowa found a larger drop in the level of one form of estrogen in women who experienced postpartum blues than in those who were not affected. While all women experience hormonal plunges, not all experience postpartum blues. It is quite possible that it is individual sensitivity to the hormone changes (rather than the measurable hormones present in the bloodstream) that causes some women, but not others, to get baby blues. This would be somewhat analogous to allergies—the determinant of who suffers hay fever is the individual's sensitivity, not the pollen or ragweed itself. Dr. O'Hara found that a history of premenstrual depression was highly correlated with baby blues, which indirectly supports the idea that individual sensitivity to hormonal drops is seen in both PMS and baby blues.

Baby blues typically goes away on its own. While many women with PPD have also had baby blues, they often report that it resolved entirely for several weeks before the PPD started. In rare cases, baby blues is extremely severe and lasts up to fourteen days. Even so, it is still called baby blues because it resolves by the second or third postpartum week. One woman who had a very severe case of baby blues said after recovering, "I would like to lobby in an effort to change the name to something much more harsh sounding, something like 'postpartum hell.'" In other words, if you have a severe case, the word blues doesn't begin to express how terrible you feel. Also, many people who do not understand what PPD is will think that PPD is just like baby blues. Here, too, if your case of PPD is called baby blues by others, blues will not begin to express how much pain you are in. We'd like to be clear about this. If you are feeling down and are worried about the way you are feeling, and these feelings are lasting past the first two to three postpartum week, it is not the blues. Feelings of sadness or anxiety or irritability that linger past this time should be brought to the attention of your healthcare provider.

## POSTPARTUM STRESS SYNDROME OR POSTPARTUM DEPRESSION?

The most common postpartum emotional reaction is what we call *postpartum stress syndrome*, also known as *adjustment disorder*, which falls between the relatively minor baby blues and the relatively severe PPD. Approximately one in five women experience postpartum stress syndrome, yet these women may get lost in the shuffle when describing postpartum adjustment reactions, because the symptoms are not as striking as in clinical depression. In postpartum stress syndrome, women are functioning fairly well and manage to get through the day with no one else noticing how awful they feel. Their inner resources are intact enough to go through the motions and take care of what needs to be done, but there is a constant sense of disappointment that interferes with feeling good about oneself and one's new role.

Consider Leslie's story:

I'm so exhausted. I have never been so tired in my life. When I get up in the middle of the night to feed the baby, I must be on automatic pilot. Sometimes I don't even know what I'm doing, and I worry constantly that I'll make some terrible mistake. And my husband is just lying there sleeping. He has to work the next day, so of course I can't disturb him, right? After all, I don't have to "work" tomorrow. All I have to do is get up two more times in the middle of the night, then get up at 6:00 a.m. to play. After that, I get to do laundry, feed her again, change diapers a few times, try to entertain her while I pile the dirty dishes in the sink, and then throw on the one pair of dirty sweatpants that I can still squeeze this horrible body into.

If I'm lucky, she'll take a nap so I can have time to cry. I can't cry in front of her—it's bad enough that I can't just take this all in stride like everyone else does; I don't want to give her a complex on top of it. And you know what? I have to do this all again tomorrow!

The phenomenon of postpartum stress syndrome is marked by feelings of anxiety and self-doubt coupled with a deep desire to be a perfect mother. These enormous expectations of being a perfect mother, perfect wife, and in control at all times, combined with very real feelings of inadequacy and helplessness, can create unbearable stress.

Imagine writing up a job description for caring for an infant. You would include the following: extremely high performance standards (basically, flawless performance expected), extremely high stakes (your child's well-being), very little control (colic, reactions to immunizations, and sleep deprivation, to name a few areas not under your control), terrible working conditions (twenty-four hours a day, seven days a week, no vacations or coffee breaks)—and all for no pay!

When viewed from this angle, it seems remarkable that any woman ever survives the postpartum period *without* postpartum stress syndrome. It is important to keep in mind that the presence of some negative feelings does not mean you have or will get PPD. Some postpartum adjustment problems are normal parts of the transition into parenthood and/or an expanded family. In some cases, postpartum stress syndrome will be worse in mothers with more than one child, because there is that much more to juggle. Then again, postpartum stress syndrome may be more severe for first-time mothers, because there are so many new things to learn about caring for an infant. With subsequent children, it is often easier to get through postpartum stress syndrome, because past experience tells you that you will achieve a new equilibrium and that the pressures of this time won't last forever.

Postpartum stress syndrome varies greatly among women, depending on the type of stress they experience and what their resources are. Some common severe stressors that increase your susceptibility to postpartum stress syndrome include illness in yourself or your child; caesarian section; closely spaced births—having a toddler to care for along with the new baby; marital separation or significant conflict with your husband*; getting a new job or moving to a new home within months of giving birth; and financial difficulties. Even without any of these stressful situations, however, the accumulation of day-to-day hassles can lead to postpartum stress syndrome.

Some women with postpartum stress syndrome go on to develop clinical depression. Other women experience postpartum stress syndrome without an associated depression. Fortunately, many of the

---

*Throughout this book, we use the term *husband* to describe your partner. We recognize that there are many ways in which families are constituted, and that single, cohabiting, separated, or lesbian women also suffer from PPD. We use *husband* because the majority of partners will be husbands.

symptoms of postpartum stress will be relieved by the same measures that help other forms of PPD. Many of the techniques we use in treatment are equally effective for depression, anxiety, and postpartum stress syndrome. Here, too, the first step is acknowledging the reality of postpartum stress, for this will help give you permission to make nurturing yourself a priority.

## Anxiety Disorders After Childbirth

### ANXIETY/PANIC DISORDER

PPD most often occurs as a primary illness—by itself, without other emotional syndromes. However, there are related anxiety disorders that can either accompany or follow PPD. Postpartum anxiety syndromes have recently been gaining more academic and clinical attention and are now understood to be a significant part of PPD. Panic disorder and obsessive-compulsive disorder (OCD) are present at a rate of about 2 percent each in the general population, and both may be first diagnosed after, or exacerbated by, childbirth.

There is considerable overlap between postpartum depression and postpartum anxiety: many women with anxiety say they have always been worriers. Thus, it is common for a woman with a history of anxiety to experience a worsening of these symptoms during the postpartum period. When that happens, women report that although they were used to living with some anxiety, it never interfered with their lives the way is does now. Many women with postpartum panic disorder feel depressed and hopeless about the panic attacks, and about one-fifth of women who have postpartum depression have one or more panic attacks. Likewise, some women with PPD become preoccupied with housecleaning or can't get certain worries out of their mind, and some women with postpartum OCD become depressed after the onset of compulsive behaviors or the obsessive and anxiety-provoking ideas. Usually the mother can pinpoint which came first.

Most women with PPD have severe anxiety symptoms, including worrying, ruminating, panic attacks, and agitation. Anxiety attacks may be secondary to PPD or may be the primary problem. Put another way, for some women, the depressive symptoms are predominant and for others, there is mostly anxiety. Interestingly, many of the biochemical and physiologic abnormalities and medical treatments are the same in both conditions. However, although similar, postpartum panic disorder and postpartum obsessive-compulsive disorder are distinct entities that may also occur without an associated PPD. They are, unquestionably, equally as distressing as PPD.

Anita's case is typical:

Anita never felt better than she did during her pregnancy. She never had morning sickness, felt energetic up to the end, and slept better than she had in years. The delivery was uneventful, and she and her husband James were ecstatic. Her first night in the hospital, just after James had gone home, she was drifting off to sleep when she was struck by what she thought must be a heart attack. Her heart pounded; she felt dizzy, couldn't breathe, and was numb in her hands. She called the nurses, then called home and left a message on the answering machine begging James to come right back. She told him she couldn't catch her breath, and something must be terribly, terribly wrong. She insisted that the hospital staff check her blood pressure and take an electrocardiogram, and she could barely be reassured that nothing "was wrong—it's just new-mother anxiety." *Nothing? She thought. Just anxiety? Really? They should be in my shoes if they think this is nothing. It feels like I'm dying.*

Review the following symptom list to see whether you may have symptoms of an anxiety disorder. The statements included in the list may be made by women with postpartum panic disorder. Look over this list and think about whether these symptoms correspond to your own feelings. In panic disorder, these symptoms occur during specific attacks that come on without warning and usually last ten to thirty minutes. The anxiety associated with these attacks can and usually does linger beyond that time.

*Anxiety/Panic Disorder Symptom Checklist*

\_\_\_\_\_ 1.  I can't catch my breath.

\_\_\_\_\_ 2.  My heart pounds, races, and/or skips a beat.

\_\_\_\_\_ 3.  My hands shake or tremble.

\_\_\_\_\_ 4.  I have stomach pains, nausea, and/or diarrhea.

\_\_\_\_\_ 5.  I get hot flashes or chills.

\_\_\_\_\_ 6.  I feel that something terrible is about to happen.

\_\_\_\_\_ 7.  I get dizzy or light-headed.

\_\_\_\_\_ 8.  Things appear "funny" or "unreal."

\_\_\_\_\_ 9.  I worry excessively about what might happen in the future.

\_\_\_\_\_ 10. I feel like I'm dying or about to have a heart attack.

\_\_\_\_\_ 11. I am afraid to leave my house or be alone, because I might have an anxiety attack and not be able to get help.

\_\_\_\_\_ 12. I feel numb or tingly in my hands and/or around my mouth.

*With all postpartum syndromes, it is important to have a medical examination, to be sure there is no physical illness causing them, as well as a clinical diagnosis by a mental-health professional.*

## POSTPARTUM OBSESSIVE COMPULSIVE DISORDER (OCD)

Marilyn has postpartum OCD:

Three weeks after Lauren was born, Marilyn was preparing dinner in the kitchen, singing and cooing to her baby, watching the news, and slicing vegetables for a stir-fry all at once. The news program mentioned a hepatitis outbreak in one of the public schools. Suddenly, Marilyn pictured Lauren in the pediatric ward of the hospital with a severe infection. She couldn't shake the idea of how vulnerable

Lauren was to germs, and she put aside her dinner preparations to scrub down the changing table, crib, and baby bath. After forty-five minutes, she was able to resume dinner preparations.

But it got worse. Soon Marilyn was spending three or four hours a day cleaning and recleaning anything that Lauren came in contact with. She boiled and reboiled bottles, nipples, and pacifiers. Fifteen minutes after changing the baby's outfit, she would begin feeling anxious: What if there are germs on her clothes? What if I didn't wash them in hot-enough water? What if I didn't use enough detergent to kill all the germs? What if I found Lauren dead in her crib, because I didn't kill all the germs? She knew this was irrational, but her anxiety kept building until she gave in to the thought. She would strip Lauren's clothes, rewash them, and give herself a few more minutes of relief from the mounting pressure. She didn't tell anyone what she was feeling, not even her husband, because she thought people would think she had completely lost her mind.

Postpartum OCD is probably the most underdetected and undertreated of the anxiety disorders that follow childbirth, in part because women are embarrassed and reluctant to reveal what they are thinking. Women are often afraid to disclose the specific nature of their thoughts, because they fear being judged, misunderstood, labeled "crazy," or—perhaps their greatest fear of all—they worry that their baby will be taken away. Another reason postpartum OCD is often misdiagnosed is that healthcare practitioners do not always ask the right questions or do not fully understand that postpartum depression is so frequently associated with severe anxiety. Postpartum depression and OCD often coexist, but many women, as well as their doctors, focus on the depressive symptoms. Yet a study at Case Western Reserve University in Cleveland found that postpartum depression is accompanied by obsessive thoughts in 57 percent of new mothers. Healthcare providers can miss symptoms of anxiety, panic, or OCD if they are only asking about depression. Recently, increased attention is being given to the importance of screening for symptoms of both anxiety and depression during the first few months following childbirth.

Studies have shown that obsessive images of having hurt one's baby were the most common symptoms of postpartum OCD. Although these recurrent mental images of harming one's much-loved baby are quite common, a woman may be terribly ashamed to admit to them, for fear that someone will believe her to be a risk to her infant. It's important to note that although these obsessive thoughts are extremely anxiety provoking, irrepressible, and persistent, they are very different from postpartum psychosis. In postpartum OCD, mothers typically know that they are having bizarre ideas and are sure that they would not hurt their baby. They have no hallucinations, no distorted thinking, and have not lost touch with reality.

### Scary Thoughts

Most people agree that a certain level of anxiety during the postpartum period is evolutionarily adaptive; after all, it has helped parents protect their babies since the beginning of time. Anxiety is an instinctive response to threatening triggers, activating the fight-or-flight response. As outlined in Karen's book, *Dropping the Baby and Other Scary Thoughts*, anxiety, accompanied by scary thoughts during the postpartum period, is common and can manifest as worry, rumination, thoughts, obsessions, misinterpretations, images, or impulses that feel inconsistent with who the mother is. They are very upsetting. Scary thoughts are intrusive, always unwanted, and can range from "Why did I have this baby?" to images of harm coming to the baby. Needless to say, these thoughts evoke high levels of distress that can be difficult for a new mom to reconcile, especially when she is sleep deprived, hormonally compromised, and utterly overloaded.

It's important to keep in mind that in addition to being a common symptom of postpartum anxiety or postpartum depression, scary thoughts are an extremely common phenomenon with all new parents. In fact, you might be surprised to learn that almost *all* new mothers and fathers experience unwanted thoughts about their babies. According to a study by Jonathan Abramowitz, 91 percent of new mothers and 88 percent of new fathers report obsessive thoughts about their baby. That's almost every single new mother!

If anxiety and scary thoughts are so common after childbirth, how do we know when they are a problem? Although the nature of scary thoughts themselves can be quite unsettling, the actual content of these thoughts (what you are thinking, what you are envisioning) is less noteworthy than the degree of distress associated with them. For example, two women might experience a similar thought such as, "What if I drop the baby down the stairs while I'm carrying him?" One woman might be briefly startled, then quickly think about something else to distract herself. The other woman might think, "Oh my god, how can I think such a terrible thing?" Then, as she pictures the baby tumbling down the steps in front of her, she panics and believes she might indeed make that happen and decides she cannot carry her baby down the steps anymore. In this way, even though the initial thought was the same, the two women experience two different levels of distress. It is the distress itself that indicates whether something needs attention in the way of treatment or support.

The good news about the high levels of distress associated with scary thoughts is that it tells us that these thoughts are anxiety-driven and are not psychotic thoughts, even though many women say they feel like they are going crazy. Bear in mind that while scary thoughts are troubling, they are not, in and of themselves, evidence of a postpartum anxiety disorder. In other words, even though a new mother may be obsessing more than usual or worrying more than her baseline level, it is only a probable case of OCD if her level of distress interferes with her ability to function normally. Postpartum OCD is characterized by obsessions that disturb a mother's ability to get through her day. With postpartum OCD, many different symptoms may manifest, but they all involve recurrent intrusive ideas or compulsive acts that cause a great deal of distress or take up a great deal of time. Remember that it's not the specific thought or idea a woman is having that is problematic. Rather, it's the degree of distress and the extent to which it impedes her ability to function.

Obsessive-Compulsive Disorder Symptom Checklist

_____ 1.  I experience certain repeated thoughts, urges, or images that I know are ridiculous and that I try to ignore or get off my mind, because they make me feel very anxious and uncomfortable (e.g., horrifying thoughts or images of harming the baby or seeing the baby harmed).

_____ 2.  I worry excessively about purposely or accidentally causing harm to my baby or someone else I love.

_____ 3.  I have extreme doubts or fears and sometimes do certain things or avoid certain things in order to prevent bad things from happening to my baby.

_____ 4.  I have always been a worrier, but now my worrying feels out of control.

_____ 5.  I often ruminate or have thoughts that race and spin around in my head.

_____ 6.  I have a fear of becoming contaminated by germs or my baby getting sick.

_____ 7.  I do certain acts in a particular way repeatedly in order to avoid feeling extremely uncomfortable (e.g., frequent washing or cleaning excessively).

_____ 8.  I am concerned about putting things in a certain order.

_____ 9.  I find I often check and recheck things.

_____ 10. Sometimes I count or touch certain items in particular ways.

_____ 11. I often repeat certain activities to ensure that I did them right or to avoid making mistakes that might endanger my baby.

_____ 12. I avoid certain things, such as knives or sharp objects, to avoid harming my baby.

_____ 13. I avoid tasks that increase my feelings of vulnerability (e.g., not bathing my baby for fear of sexually abusing my baby).

_____ 14. I worry excessively that I do not love my baby or that my baby does not love me.

## POSTPARTUM POST-TRAUMATIC STRESS DISORDER

Postpartum post-traumatic stress disorder (PTSD) is an emotional syndrome that is triggered by a highly traumatic experience that resulted in extreme fear, helplessness, or terror. The symptoms are classified in three clusters:

1. Intrusive memories, thoughts, flashbacks, and/or dreams of the event
2. Avoidance of reminders, or a general sense of emotional numbing
3. Physiological overactivity, as manifested by angry outbursts, hyperactive startle responses (fight-or-flight reactions or panic attacks in response to environmental cues that remind you of the trauma), or constantly being on guard

Women who have recently given birth may experience postpartum PTSD from one of two sources. The first of these is a childbirth-related trauma, in which you or your baby's life was in danger. Childbirth-related trauma may include events such as an emergency cesarean section, fetal distress, emergency resuscitation of your newborn, or other maternal or infant life-threatening conditions.

New mothers with past traumatic experiences and a history of PTSD from non-childbirth-related causes may also find that having a baby triggers a major flare-up of PTSD. The most common cause of PTSD in women is sexual trauma: sexual abuse, rape, attempted rape, or incest. Other causes of PTSD in women include physical abuse (in childhood or domestic violence), car accidents, and military service.

The reasons that childbirth can trigger flare-ups of previous PTSD are complex. One factor is that giving birth involves being physically vulnerable, immobilized to a certain extent, and dependent on others, which may be experienced by victimized women as a trigger for intrusive memories. Being hooked up to an IV or a fetal monitor, unable to get out of bed after a Cesarean section, and feeling overwhelmed by pain and fear can be very reminiscent of many traumatic events. Another huge factor is the emotional vulnerability of becoming a new mother. Seeing the helplessness and neediness of a newborn may cause the mother to identify with her own baby—perhaps needy and helpless is just how she felt during an abusive relationship, for example. Some mothers feel a vicarious terror on behalf of their defenseless new baby—afraid that someone they love more than anything could be hurt, too. These feelings can temporarily open the floodgates for intrusive thoughts, excessive vigilance, anxiety attacks, and insomnia that had previously been under control.

*Postpartum PTSD Checklist*

_____ 1. I have experienced one or more severe psychological traumas in the past.

_____ 2. I have repeated distressing thoughts or images of the traumatic events.

_____ 3. I have flashbacks about the trauma.

_____ 4. I avoid triggers that may remind me of the trauma.

_____ 5. Just thinking about the trauma makes my heart race.

_____ 6. I am always watching out to try to protect myself and my loved ones from trauma.

_____ 7. My anger gets the best of me, and sometimes I lash out at people I love over trivial things.

_____ 8. I don't feel like myself since the trauma.

## What Is a Postpartum Emergency?

Postpartum emergencies are, fortunately, very rare. Unfortunately, the rarest postpartum disorder (*postpartum psychosis*, present in one or two per thousand deliveries) and its extremely rare tragic outcome (harm to a child) are sensationalized in the media and massively overemphasized relative to the common forms of PPD. In reality, the most common serious risk of PPD is suicide, not infanticide.

Because a delay in getting help in postpartum emergencies may have very serious consequences, we are including a list of symptoms that includes those that signal the need for immediate intervention. Some are symptoms of postpartum psychosis, in which hallucinations or delusions accompany other symptoms. If you suspect that you may have postpartum psychosis, you should immediately contact your doctor. A "yes" response to *any* of the symptoms below means you need to be aggressive about seeking help from a professional. Get help *today* if your own feelings match any of these symptoms or if you have any doubt about your ability to keep yourself and others safe.

*Postpartum Emergency Symptom Checklist*

_____ 1.  I am afraid that I might harm myself in order to escape this pain.

_____ 2.  I am afraid that I might actually do something to hurt my baby.

_____ 3.  I hear sounds or voices when no one is around.

_____ 4.  I do not feel that my thoughts are my own or that they are totally in my control.

_____ 5.  I am being controlled by forces beyond myself.

_____ 6.  I have not slept at all in forty-eight hours or more.

_____ 7.  I do not feel loving toward my baby and can't even go through the motions of taking care of him/her.

_____ 8.  I am rapidly losing weight without trying to.

Keep in mind: most women with PPD have no emergency symptoms and are never at risk of hurting themselves or anyone else. If you are not certain, a mental-health professional can help you sort this out. Women with postpartum psychosis have a biologic crisis, which must be treated immediately. This book should not be used until medical intervention is underway. Once the psychosis has significantly resolved, this book may be helpful.

## How to Use This Book

You may be wondering where to go from here. What can you do about PPD* when you or someone you love experiences it? How do you get through it? How can you endure the emotional pain and still manage to nurture yourself back to your old self again? What can you do if your wife, daughter, sister, neighbor, or daughter-in-law is suffering from PPD? The first decision you must make is how you plan to recover. We have organized this book along the avenue of recovery that we commonly see in our practices and in our discussions with women who have recovered from PPD without professional help. The typical pattern of recovery is as follows:

FIRST, try to use your internal resources to support yourself as much as possible. In mild cases, this alleviates some symptoms, and women will often move straight to the third step. When PPD is more severe, those who continue to feel significant pain must consider the second step, seeking professional help.

SECOND, turn to a professional if the illness is not responding to your attempts to recover. Most women put off seeking professional help until they have tried to get better on their own. Some women, especially those who have been treated by a mental-health professional in the past, immediately turn to a therapist as the first step. In some

---

*We will assume that you have confirmed this diagnosis for the remainder of this book.

cases, the decision to seek professional help is based on symptom severity. Women who are in severe distress should consider starting at step two and returning to the first step after some early symptom relief is under way. Again, any reader who has any of the emergency symptoms should immediately contact a professional. Once step two has helped you master step one, you are ready for the third step.

THIRD, turn to those around you to help you make it through this crisis. Many women with PPD are far more comfortable at giving support than they are at taking it from family and friends. That is why this step comes after you have done what you can to make it on your own, to quiet the nagging feeling that "I should be able to handle this myself." After you master this step, you are ready for the introspection that comes in the late stages of PPD recovery.

FOURTH, begin to examine, acknowledge, grieve, and move beyond the losses that a mother with PPD typically experiences. The losses that most mothers go through, which are often exaggerated in PPD, involve unmet fantasies about what motherhood would be like, major changes in your relationship with your partner, and loss of autonomy that comes from the necessity of putting another person's needs first. PPD may ignite smoldering issues with your own parents, and we will explore in Chapter 13 some of the intergenerational issues that are pertinent to PPD.

FINALLY, look ahead. We address many of the common concerns that women who have recovered from PPD have as they try to sort through what having emerged from this illness means.

We do not expect you to read this book in a single sitting and recover within a few days. We have tried to keep the material brief and focused on particular issues. Use this book in any way that meets your needs. If you can only read a chapter at a time, fine. On other days, or at another time in the day, you might find yourself motivated to do more. Do as little or as much as you find helpful.

We strongly encourage you to use all the resources you have to help you recover. This includes mustering your strength and also being receptive to all the possibilities around you—your husband, your family, his family, your family doctor, a psychiatrist, a therapist, medication, the new-mother's group at your church or synagogue, and the local PPD self-help group, to name a few. It is really and truly okay to ask for and receive help from others. *You will get better. You will feel like yourself again.* Right now, you need to accept this emotional pain and try to stop pretending it will go away by itself. If you are in treatment, we urge you to use this book in conjunction with your therapist or doctor. Your therapist can help by clarifying those issues that are especially significant to your individual situation.

Remember, the road to recovery is not smooth. There will be some good days and some bad days. Eventually, the number of good hours in a day will increase. Then, the number of good days will increase.

Be patient. Take one day at a time, and we will help you get through this.

# ···[ 2 ]···

# "I'M MAKING MYSELF CRAZY"

## *Breaking Negative Thought Patterns*

S UPPOSE YOU ARE ON YOUR WAY to your six-week checkup and
you find yourself in a terrible traffic jam on the highway. There
is no way off, no way out. Your appointment is in fifteen minutes,
and since you haven't been feeling well, you are anxious to get there
on time. There was no way to anticipate this tie-up. So you start to
think:

> What if I miss my appointment? I'll probably have to wait two more
> months before I can make another one. I'm sure I'll get charged for
> missing this appointment. What if something is really wrong with
> me? I have to go to make sure everything's okay.

Then, you begin to experience some physical signs of anxiety: your
breathing becomes rapid, your chest tightens, you can feel your heart
palpitating, your stomach begins to hurt. Now you think:

I can't breathe. I knew there was something wrong with me! What if something happens to me out here? Would I stop strangers in their cars? They would think I'm crazy. What if I needed to get to a hospital? Not even an ambulance could get through this! How would I get help?

Here we see an example of how quickly negative thinking can get out of control. Spontaneous thought patterns like these are very common when you have PPD. Fortunately, there has been very successful psychological research on "think traps" that has yielded some useful therapeutic techniques. Much of what we will discuss here is based on the fundamental elements of cognitive therapy, as developed by Aaron Beck and David Burns. Their work was particularly revolutionary, because it was based on the notion that people could actually control and change the way they feel.

You will learn that negative thinking and thought distortions are actually symptoms of PPD. As with any symptom of an illness, there are things you can do to make it better and things you can do to make it worse. Learning to change the way you think about and respond to certain situations can have a direct impact on the way you feel. In our practices, we rely on this basic principle of cognitive therapy to help control the emotional bombardment that most women with PPD feel.

## How Not to Become Your Own Worst Enemy

As you learn about these cognitive principles, you will see how, inadvertently, you may be getting in the way of your recovery. In the early phases of PPD, women tend to get lost in a pattern of repetitive negative thoughts. We have listed some of the statements we often hear women say about having PPD that actually serve to reinforce how poorly they are feeling. Read over these statements and check any or all of them that apply to how you feel right now about having PPD:

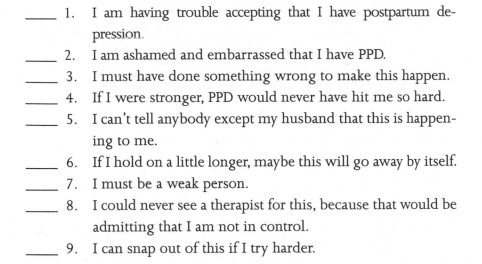

\_\_\_\_ 1. I am having trouble accepting that I have postpartum depression.

\_\_\_\_ 2. I am ashamed and embarrassed that I have PPD.

\_\_\_\_ 3. I must have done something wrong to make this happen.

\_\_\_\_ 4. If I were stronger, PPD would never have hit me so hard.

\_\_\_\_ 5. I can't tell anybody except my husband that this is happening to me.

\_\_\_\_ 6. If I hold on a little longer, maybe this will go away by itself.

\_\_\_\_ 7. I must be a weak person.

\_\_\_\_ 8. I could never see a therapist for this, because that would be admitting that I am not in control.

\_\_\_\_ 9. I can snap out of this if I try harder.

If you checked any one of these statements, you are thinking in a self-defeating manner that may interfere with your efforts to feel better. If you checked two or more (and it is common to check all nine), you are definitely standing in your own way. To appreciate the direct impact these negative thoughts have on how you feel, pick any one of them and repeat it to yourself over and over. For instance, pick number 4: "If I were stronger, PPD would never have hit me so hard. If I were stronger, PPD would never have hit me so hard. If I were stronger . . . " Soon the phrase takes on a life of its own, like a mantra, and you can't help beginning to feel weak and depressed.

When you have PPD, negative thoughts are usually so automatic they barely enter your consciousness; like elevator music, they drone on in the background. If you can replace those thoughts with realistic ones, it will break the negative cycle and help you come to terms with what you are feeling. Here are some examples of thoughts you can substitute for those statements that you checked earlier that relate to having PPD. Try these positive affirmations instead:

1. I have postpartum depression.
2. What I am feeling are symptoms of this illness. I am not making this up.
3. Bleak as life seems now, this pain will not last forever.
4. I am not going crazy.
5. This is a real illness, and it can be treated.
6. I didn't do anything to make this happen.
7. This is not my fault.
8. I may have bad days, and I will have some good days. I will not always feel like this.
9. I can choose to be active in the course of my recovery and help myself feel better.

As you read these affirmations, try to be aware of how each one makes you feel. For example, read number 7 again: "This is not my fault." Most women experiencing PPD are quite hard on themselves and believe that its presence implies a moral weakness or some character flaw. It is easy to understand where these feelings come from when you consider how our society has traditionally viewed emotional illness.

When you repeat "This is not my fault" several times, does it soothe you in some small way? Can you begin to believe that PPD is really not your fault and that you did nothing to make this happen? If this does not come naturally to you, try repeating the phrase a few times a day. Write "This is not my fault" on index cards and stick them to the refrigerator, the bathroom mirror, the kitchen sink. Read this phrase throughout your day. It may sound too simple, but repeatedly exposing yourself to the words really will help. After a while, you will begin to absorb the thought at a deeper level.

## Distorted Self-Perceptions

When you have PPD, it is understandably easy to criticize yourself or to become completely preoccupied with negative thoughts. This is a classic self-fulfilling prophecy: think enough negative thoughts, and you will indeed feel worse. Earlier, we looked at negative statements pertaining to PPD, the illness. Now let's look at negative statements that relate to how you feel about yourself. Read the following statements and check those that seem to influence the way you feel about yourself since your baby was born:

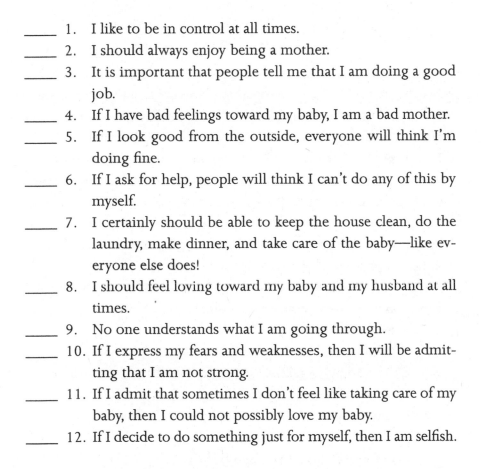

_____ 1. I like to be in control at all times.

_____ 2. I should always enjoy being a mother.

_____ 3. It is important that people tell me that I am doing a good job.

_____ 4. If I have bad feelings toward my baby, I am a bad mother.

_____ 5. If I look good from the outside, everyone will think I'm doing fine.

_____ 6. If I ask for help, people will think I can't do any of this by myself.

_____ 7. I certainly should be able to keep the house clean, do the laundry, make dinner, and take care of the baby—like everyone else does!

_____ 8. I should feel loving toward my baby and my husband at all times.

_____ 9. No one understands what I am going through.

_____ 10. If I express my fears and weaknesses, then I will be admitting that I am not strong.

_____ 11. If I admit that sometimes I don't feel like taking care of my baby, then I could not possibly love my baby.

_____ 12. If I decide to do something just for myself, then I am selfish.

This list is just the beginning. We suspect that you can easily continue and add your own list of distorted thoughts that get in the way of your feeling good about yourself. Complete the following with some additional distorted thoughts regarding your expectations of being a mother:

1. _____
2. _____
3. _____
4. _____
5. _____

## Replacing Distorted Thoughts with Positive Statements

Because recognizing that you have negative thoughts is a lot easier than replacing them with positive ones, we have provided you with some examples of positive thoughts to use while working toward recovery. Read over the statements listed below. Copy one of the statements onto a Post-it or index card and spend some time thinking about what that idea means to you. If you can, try to talk it over with someone who cares for you—your husband, mother, or therapist. Post the statement on the refrigerator. Go back and look at it as often as you need to. When you are feeling especially bad, anxious, or pessimistic, practice saying it to yourself. There is no right or wrong number of times to do this—you will find the right pace for yourself. Then, repeat the process tomorrow with a new positive statement.

1. I'm doing the best I can.
2. This is going to take a long time, whether or not I try to speed it up. I must take one day at a time.
3. I cannot expect too much from myself right now.
4. It is okay to make mistakes.
5. There will be good days and bad days.
6. It is okay for me to have negative feelings. If I fight having these feelings, it might take longer to feel better.
7. Even though I feel so bad, just getting through the day is proof of my strength. I can be proud of how much I have accomplished when I get through the day feeling this bad.

8. I know that some of the pain I am feeling right now is part of the recovery process.

9. Today, when I am feeling bad, I know that I will not feel bad all of the time. This is just a bad day. I will get through this day the best I can. I will try to rest. I will pamper myself a bit. I will treat myself well, because I deserve it. And I will wait this out.

10. Some of what I am feeling is just like what other mothers feel. Not all of my bad feelings are symptoms of PPD. All mothers of new babies feel tired, irritable, or stressed at times.

11. It's okay that not everyone understands what I am going through. I still have a real illness that is treatable, even if other people don't know anything about PPD.

12. I will feel like myself again.

Remember that it is important to repeat these statements, even if you have trouble believing them right now. You are in the process of internalizing them, and it will take some time. Nevertheless, the best way to undo negative thinking is to replace it with new positive ideas. As you repeat each statement over and over, it becomes more likely that this new belief will become automatic instead of the previous, mistaken one.

## Anxiety and Depression: Cycles of Despair

Depressed and anxious feelings are excruciatingly painful. By themselves, these feelings are terrible to experience for any period of time. However, something even worse happens with these feelings when an emotional syndrome sets in—they trigger thoughts and behaviors that lead to a downward spiral in which the depression and anxiety cause more depressed feelings, attitudes, beliefs, and thoughts:

I feel sad. Therefore . . .

I cannot keep these sad feelings away, no matter how hard I try.
   Therefore . . .

I am helpless about these sad feelings. Therefore . . .

I am helpless about other things. Therefore . . .

I am helpless about everything. Therefore . . .

I am a failure because I am helpless. Therefore . . .

I am a failure as a mother because I am helpless. Therefore . . .

I am a failure as a person because I am a failure as a mother.
   Therefore . . .

I am a total failure. Therefore . . .

I feel sad about being a total failure.


You can easily see how the cycle starts over, getting progressively
worse with each turn. The original thought—I feel sad—is lost in the
spiral of despair. This is what we call a positive-feedback loop—the
end product feeds back into the loop, perpetuating and intensifying
the original feeling of sadness.

A similar positive-feedback cycle occurs in postpartum anxiety:


I feel anxious. Therefore . . .

I might have another anxiety attack. Therefore . . .

I can start to feel my heart beat faster just thinking about having
   an anxiety attack. Therefore . . .

Now my heart is skipping beats. Therefore . . .

I might have a heart disease that no doctor can diagnose.
   Therefore . . .

I am starting to hyperventilate. Therefore . . .

I can't catch my breath at all now. Therefore . . .

Something terrible is going to happen to me. Therefore . . .

I am out of control. Therefore . . .

I will never feel normal again. Therefore . . .

Now I am really panicked about knowing I will never feel normal again.

Again, the cycle spirals downward. The original feeling of anxiety gets worse through secondary anxiety, and the anxious feelings slide into a cycle of despair. The anxious feelings trigger physical sensations, which in turn trigger more anxiety.

## Secondary Automatic Thoughts: "What If? . . ."

Within these cycles, secondary automatic thoughts perpetuate more despair. These are self-defeating, self-criticizing thoughts that immediately follow the original feeling. They tend to come in certain patterns, with two of the most common patterns being catastrophizing (e.g., this anxious feeling must mean that I will have a heart attack) and overgeneralizing (e.g., because I am powerless over my sad feelings right now, I am totally powerless over my sad feelings forever and ever). Catastrophizing occurs when we follow a painful feeling with the thought, "What if this feeling turns into a catastrophe?" When we overgeneralize, we assume that the way we are feeling about a specific situation applies to every situation at all times. Catastrophizing and overgeneralizing share a tendency to carry thoughts to a black-or-white extreme—to always see the half-full cup as almost irrevocably empty. Remember that both of these patterns may not be a part of your everyday thought process—they may be present only as a function of these downward spirals.

## Identifying Your Own Secondary Automatic Thoughts

The first step toward understanding how this cycle of despair can be interrupted is to get back in touch with the original feeling that precipitated the cycle. After a particularly painful episode, such as a panic attack or a period of severe crying, think back to what was happening right before the episode. What were you doing? Feeling? Thinking?

*Just before* I felt so overwhelmed, I was

_____

*Just before* I felt so overwhelmed, I began to feel

_____

*Just before* I felt so overwhelmed, I began to think

_____

*While* I was feeling overwhelmed, I was thinking

_____

*After* it was over, I realized that

_____


After identifying the original feeling, your objective is to prevent yourself from having the secondary automatic thoughts: In looking back, were there secondary fears and worries that you might have been able to interrupt? Were there things that you began to feel and/or think that developed after the original feeling of anxiety or sadness? Think about the previous example of being late for a doctor's appointment. For many people in this situation, the original feeling would be frustration, impatience, or anxiety. But as we can see from our example, one of the earliest negative thoughts that got you off track was, "What if something is really wrong with me?"

The fear that there could be a medical problem that would not get attended to if the appointment was missed was enough to generate the physical manifestations of anxiety. "What if something physical is really wrong with me" is an example of an automatic thought for many people prone to anxiety. This is the point where you need to learn how to spot these thoughts and counter them with a positive statement such as, "There is probably nothing else wrong with me. I've really felt okay lately. If I miss the appointment, I can probably reschedule soon enough." The trick is catching the automatic thought at the earliest point in order for the intervention to be effective. If you recognize the secondary automatic thoughts that you reveal to yourself, you will often be able to interrupt the feedback cycle that anxiety and depression cause.

This awareness will enable you to have more control over your thoughts. Plan ahead by trying to anticipate the automatic negative thoughts that follow painful feelings. ("I hate traffic jams. I know this will make me nervous. I always think I feel sick when I'm nervous. This will probably happen now, too.") Be prepared to use logic in your positive statements to avoid amplifying a specific fear into a generalized state of anxiety. This may sound like an impossible task in the midst of an anxiety attack, but the more you practice it, the easier it will become.

## Breaking the Cycle

Using the two earlier examples of downward spirals, let's look more closely at how you can interrupt the cycle of negative thinking. After the very first negative thought, immediately insert a positive statement before a secondary automatic thought has a chance to enter and precipitate a spiral of despair:

> I feel sad. Also . . .
> I cannot keep myself from having sad feelings right now. But . . .
> I remember times when I have not felt as sad as I feel right now.
>   Therefore . . .
> I am only powerless over my sad feelings for the moment. So . . .
> It is not a catastrophe to have sad feelings right now. Therefore . . .
> I will accept these sad feelings, but only for right now.

If your negative thoughts begin to spiral downward, insert a positive one at the earliest opportunity:

I am feeling anxious. Therefore . . .

I might have another anxiety attack. Therefore . . .

I can start to feel my heart beat faster just thinking about having an anxiety attack. However . . .

This is only an anxiety attack. Therefore . . .

Although I feel terrible and I feel terrified, I am okay physically. Also . . .

I have *always* survived an anxiety attack, no matter how terrible and terrified I felt during it. Therefore . . .

I will survive this anxiety attack. Therefore . . .

I am only powerless over my anxiety for the moment. So . . .

It is not a catastrophe to have anxiety right now. Therefore . . .

I will accept this anxiety, but only for right now.

## The Exit Ramp

Let's return to our original positive-feedback highway loop. As the traffic crawls forward, you notice an exit ramp ahead to the right. You are not sure where that will take you, but you are certain you will feel better if you can just get off the highway. You ease your way out of the flow of traffic and move onto the shoulder. As you approach the exit, you notice your heartbeat has slowed down. Your breathing has relaxed a bit. Now you think:

I'm definitely going to be late. There is nothing I can do about it now. I'll be okay. I just have to figure out how to get there from this direction and explain why I'm so late when I arrive.

Knowing that you have an option is a very important concept for you to remember if you suffer from anxiety symptoms. Often, the anxiety comes from a feeling of being trapped in some way, either physically or emotionally. Catastrophizing and overgeneralizing are responses to this entrapment. Most of the time, your tendency to exaggerate the outcome of a situation is a habit you have developed. You are used to thinking this way under stress. In order to unlearn these patterns of thinking, you have to replace the habit with new information.

Finding an exit ramp means helping yourself find a way out of an anxiety-provoking situation. If there isn't an obvious alternative route, you'll have to make one up for yourself by working out some solutions or options that are acceptable to you. In the example of the traffic jam, if there had not been an exit ramp, one of your options might have been to leave your car on the shoulder and walk to your destination or to the nearest stopping point. We are not suggesting that this would be the most productive option or that you even have to act on it. What we are suggesting is that sometimes, for some people, *just knowing they have an option out* gives them the leeway they need to manage their anxiety enough to get them through the situation. In other words, although you may not actually get out of your car and walk, knowing that you *can* if you choose to may make you feel calm enough to sit out the traffic jam.

## Evolutionary Instincts

Remember Anita, who experienced a panic attack in the hospital after the birth of her child? After calling her husband for comfort and re-assurance, she felt well for the remainder of her hospital stay. But the anxiety attacks recurred after she and the new baby came home from the hospital. Friends tried to reassure her, "It's just baby blues. It will go away." This seemed to get her through a few days, but then she had two more attacks over the next week. She saw her obstetrician for a physical exam, and all seemed fine. He laughed when Anita asked if she had a heart condition, saying, "Heart condition? You? Don't be silly—you just came through the obstetric equivalent of the Boston Marathon. Giving birth is like an advanced treadmill test, and believe me, your cardiovascular system passed the test."

Anita was temporarily reassured and was able to ignore the twinges of chest pain and palpitations she felt now and then. But shortly thereafter, just before falling asleep, she had a full-blown attack. She had now suffered for three weeks with these attacks and began to feel depressed, often crying about the thought that these attacks could plague her for the rest of her life. She called her obstetrician again, this time in tears. Her doctor suggested she might have postpartum depression and referred her to a therapist.

Anita's therapist realized that the depression had set in after the occurrence of several anxiety attacks. She explained that Anita's conviction that something dreadful was about to happen to her each time she had an attack was caused by the age-old fight-or-flight response, left over from the time when life was very dangerous due to constant threats of attack by animals, warring tribes, or natural disasters. In those days, infants whose mothers had very sensitive "radar" for dangerous conditions were the most likely to survive. These mothers' fight-or-flight responses prepared them either to flee the danger or to fight the attacker. Although there were no wild animals in Anita's comfortable suburban townhouse, and her easily triggered fight-or-flight response was not needed to ensure her family's safety, she was experiencing a similar primal instinct in response to fear.

Anita felt relieved by learning what was happening to her, and she kept a journal of her attacks from early symptoms of anxiety to full-blown panic. She caught herself automatically assuming that her physical symptoms were a sign of imminent danger. She learned to counteract her catastrophizing with reassuring phrases, including, "This anxiety will not hurt me. I will be okay once this anxiety passes. This feeling is just anxiety and not evidence of something worse." Gradually, she was able to see the connection between her protective maternal instincts and how they triggered a particularly strong fight-or-flight response. She continued to have occasional uncomfortable but mild anxiety attacks, but after learning to interrupt her catastrophizing, she had no more frightening episodes.

## Choosing to Change

The concept of breaking negative thought patterns is based on the belief that you have a great deal of power over how you feel at certain times. As we have noted, people actually behave or think in ways that reinforce their anxious or depressed feelings. To illustrate further, consider the following: If you knew that doing a certain thing would help make you feel better, why would you not choose to do it, or at least try it?

There are a couple of reasons why women with PPD may not be able to put forth the effort to change these patterns: You may be too tired, anxious, or depressed to activate a change. If you are used to responding with anxiety to a certain situation, it becomes a habitual response. As with any bad habit, there is some level of comfort with what is familiar to you. It may seem as though the extra energy needed to change this response is not worth it, but holding on to your anxiety actually increases your tension and allows the cycle to continue.

Here are five suggestions to help you cope with anxiety attacks. It may be very hard to make yourself follow them at first, but don't give up! It gets easier the more you practice. And remember, every anxiety attack will come to an end.

**1. Be Aware:** Be aware of the situations that provoke anxiety reactions or other mood changes. Try to identify triggers that elicit these habitual responses. Bringing these thoughts to your awareness level can actually promote change all by itself.

**2. Stop It:** Recognize this response pattern and just tell yourself to STOP. Wear a rubber band around your wrist. Snap it (hard!) when you begin to feel a panic attack coming on or when you notice you are obsessing or thinking in a self-defeating manner.

Visualize the word STOP in letters that you dress up. Start by picturing the letter S. Add a hat or scarf, a sweater, and a skirt. Add shoes. Next picture the letter T. Dress the letter in a fancy dress, high heels, and a necklace. Complete this exercise for O and P. Then visualize the entire word *STOP* in your mind as you have dressed it.

**3. Distract Yourself:** Find something that can replace this old habit, even if only for the moment. Take a walk, call a friend, count the number of tiles on the floor. Or try counting objects: for example, look around the room and count everything that is blue or that starts with the letter T. This is especially useful when you have an older child and can make this exercise a game to be played together. She or he won't need to know that you are having an anxiety attack.

Some women use a technique called progressive relaxation. In this exercise, you lie down with your eyes closed and progressively tense up and then relax your muscles. You start at the head by tightening your forehead muscles for a slow count of five, followed by release of those same muscles for a count of five. Then tense your cheeks and jaw for a count of five, followed by a release for five counts. Move down to your neck, shoulders, arms and fists, chest, abdomen, hips, thighs, calves, ankles. (Be aware that a subgroup of women with anxiety cannot do this, because muscle relaxation increases their feeling of vulnerability. Simply stop if this happens to you.)

**4. Give Yourself Options:** Give yourself permission to escape an anxiety-provoking situation ("I can excuse myself and leave the meeting if I'm too nervous"). Remember, this doesn't mean you will actually do it. But by giving yourself the option to, and permission to, you will feel better.

**5. Support Your Choices:** "If I do have to leave the meeting, that will be okay. It's not the worst thing in the world. I'm sure I'm not the first person who has ever done that!"

# "I Just Want This to Go Away"

*Putting Feelings First and Accepting Postpartum Depression*

> *Right away, I knew something was going on. I didn't feel like myself anymore. I felt confused and uncertain. My doctor said maybe I had postpartum depression, but I'm not that kind of person. Besides, I felt like something else was terribly wrong. I couldn't eat. I couldn't sleep. I felt so scared and lonely. I tried so hard to pretend I wasn't feeling that way. It seemed like the more I tried to make it go away, the worse I felt.*
>
> —JANET, PPD SUPPORT-GROUP PARTICIPANT

*I*F YOU RECOGNIZED YOURSELF in any of the descriptions of PPD from Chapter 1, you are one step closer to understanding that you have PPD. Seeing the diagnosis on paper and identifying it is the easy part. The hard part is accepting it in your heart. The process of recovery will move along more quickly when you are able to accept, on an emotional level, what is happening to you.

As you keep in mind some of the positive statements from Chapter 2, you are probably noticing that a lot of what you are being asked to do here is much easier said than done. We know this is true. But part of what makes it so difficult to accept that you have PPD and believe what you are saying when you repeat these statements is due to the emotional responses you are having.

As with most psychological disorders, there is an unfortunate stigma attached to PPD that contributes to denial in many women: "Don't worry about me, I'll snap out of this. There's nothing wrong with me." Denial and the anger that usually accompanies it are common, almost knee-jerk reactions to being told you have PPD. Early stages of denial are not only understandable; they may also be helpful defenses. Denial is what makes it possible for you to continue to do things you don't feel like doing, such as cleaning the house, going to work, getting the children dressed. But when denial is carried too far, the mechanism that originally set out to protect you backfires and can delay the healing process. This, coupled with the anger that is associated with early stages of denial, prevents you from taking care of yourself. Working through your denial is an essential first step toward acceptance of PPD. And with this acceptance come relief and the first hint of light at the end of the tunnel.

## Beginning to Accept PPD

"It's Not Fair!"

One of the hardest obstacles to overcome is your notion that it is not fair that you have PPD. Preoccupation with the unfairness of having PPD is a common form of denial in the early stages of discovering that you have it. It isn't fair that it happened to you and not to your neighbor down the street. It isn't fair that so many other women seem to have babies with little or no difficulties.

Lynn is twenty-seven years old and has just had her first baby. She is wondering why she feels so badly all the time.

I have two friends who just had babies this month. One of them is married to an alcoholic husband who never comes home until the middle of the night, and the other friend didn't even want to get pregnant! They are both happy as can be. They go out together and take their babies to the park, and all I seem to do is sit around worrying about how bad I feel. Having PPD stinks!

Lynn is in denial to some extent. Her anger serves to block out the grief that she's fighting so hard to avoid. Even though she says she has PPD, she is focusing on how much better off everyone else is as a way of not thinking about her own problem. Unfortunately, by constantly complaining about how unfair it is, she is preventing herself from going beyond mere intellectual acknowledgment of her condition, which she will need to do to recover.

Think about someone who has diabetes. It's not fair that she has to restrict her diet. It's not fair that she has to give herself shots of insulin. It's not fair that she can't eat that piece of cake. But if she spends too much time resenting how unfair life is, she may not give herself the insulin that she needs, or she may eat that piece of cake, or she may behave in ways that are contraindicated for her illness. In this way, her denial interferes with her taking the steps necessary to improve her situation. Likewise, if you are to recover from PPD, you simply have to tell yourself that this is what you have, fair or not.

## Letting Someone Else Know How You Feel

Some women know they are beginning to accept that they have PPD when they are able to tell someone else about it. Consider Susie, who thought that if she waited long enough, she would eventually get better, and she wouldn't have to tell anyone how she had been feeling:

Some months after her baby was born, Susie made plans to have lunch with her close friend, Dana. She postponed the date as long as possible, hoping that she would feel better. Dana has two children of her own and always seems to do everything right. She looks great, has something nice to say to everyone, and dresses as though she stepped right out of a fashion magazine. Susie looks at herself in the mirror and sees a tired face and sad expression. She has been trying to fake it, but she is getting fed up with pretending she is fine. She feels ashamed and alone.

When she meets Dana and hugs her in greeting, Susie is tempted to let down her guard ever so slightly, just enough to let someone reach out and help her. Although she feels embarrassed, she knows she needs to tell Dana how she has been feeling.

Over lunch, Susie shares details of her depression: the long, tedious mornings; the tearful afternoons; the anxiety attacks. Dana listens quietly, then casually shares the story of how she, too, experienced a similar episode after the birth of her first child. She took antidepressants for a period of time and has kept most of her experience a secret from her friends, just as Susie has been doing.

It feels great for both of them finally to talk about it. Susie is relieved and somewhat surprised to hear that Dana was depressed—she always looked so upbeat and composed from the outside. But then again, Susie thinks, so do I! Talking about it makes them feel so much better—they can't believe they waited so long to do it.

Susie sees that Dana's symptoms are gone now and that she is feeling well. Susie feels hopeful about her PPD for the first time.

In this case, we see how, in her early phase of acceptance, Susie risks talking to a friend, and in doing so, finds support and reassurance. Dana feels well again, and so will she. Realizing that Dana has completely recovered from the misery Susie is experiencing suddenly puts it in perspective for her: *she has an illness with symptoms.* These symptoms will eventually resolve when the illness is gone.

There will be people who understand what you are going through and people who will not. We recall one woman who finally decided to tell her friend how badly she was feeling and was devastated by her friend's response: "When my kids were little, I didn't have time for all that! You're lucky you have time to get depressed!"

Because the symptoms of PPD can be vague and easily misunderstood, some women who reach out and let others know how they are feeling become frustrated by misinformed friends, family members, and professionals who often give contradictory advice: "Don't worry, you just had a baby. Everything will be fine"; or "Just relax. If you're nervous, you'll have a nervous baby!" "Have a glass of wine, you'll feel better"; or "You're just not busy enough. You have too much time to think. Get a hobby."

> Amy decided to tell her mother-in-law about the difficulty she had been having with PPD. She made a tentative first step: "I have PPD. Have you ever heard of it?" Her mother-in-law responded with a resounding, "PPD, that's ridiculous. I hope you snap out of it soon. You have a family to take care of, you know!" Amy was confident enough in her own acceptance of her PPD not to let her mother-in-law's reaction upset her. Whether or not her mother-in-law was capable of understanding the situation, Amy felt it was important for her to know. Amy quickly learned to set limits and only tell her mother-in-law relevant information about her PPD, such as, "I'm having a bad day. I need such and such from you today." She also talked to her husband and hoped that he would be able to help by further explaining the situation to his mother.

It is never easy to decide whether or not to tell someone what you are going through. It can be a tough judgment call, and you may need to make some careful choices about with whom to share your feelings. But as we saw in Susie's story, sometimes telling someone can also bring welcome relief and support. We feel it is very important to share how you are feeling with someone you trust. If you are more comfortable sharing in an anonymous setting, a PPD support group might be helpful. You must go at your own pace and decide for yourself when is the right time and who is the right person. You will know when you are ready.

If, like Amy, you tell someone about having PPD and that person says something stupid, hurtful, or just doesn't get it, you don't need to give her the power to move you back a stage in your own acceptance. We have treated many women who have successfully recovered from PPD without having close friends or family members validate their illness.

## Identifying and Understanding Your Feelings

Once you begin to accept that PPD is a real illness, you can begin to understand that many of the feelings you are experiencing are symptoms. Often, women in our practices say to us, "Yes, I know I have PPD, but why can't I sleep? Why does my heart pound? Why do I feel so out of sorts? Why can't I just stop feeling sad, when I know I should be happy?"

We see this kind of thinking as a sign of denial of PPD, even though on the surface it seems that the woman understands her condition. In other words, preoccupation with painful feelings and painful physical sensations signals only a superficial acceptance. For example, imagine someone saying, "I know I have bronchitis, but why am I coughing so much? Why can't I just stop hurting in my chest?" We would conclude that person has not truly accepted having bronchitis. Otherwise, she would recognize the symptoms of bronchitis as just that. If she doesn't recognize her symptoms for what they are, she may not follow the recommended treatment or may waste time and energy trying to find an alternative explanation for them.

Tremendous relief and hope come from recognizing that the emotional and physical pain you are experiencing are symptoms. If you cannot accept at a deep level that these ancillary effects are part of PPD, you will be unable to look forward to a complete recovery. One mother put it this way: "Until I realized that I had PPD, I just thought this was how my life was going to be now that I was a mother."

It is easier for people to accept physical changes as evidence of an illness, and because emotional changes are invisible, they can be more easily dismissed. There is no diagnostic test to provide physical proof of a PPD diagnosis. However, it is important for you to understand that it is, nonetheless, a real illness, and like any physical ailment, it has specific symptoms. Below, we have listed some of the most common physical symptoms of PPD:

*Physical Symptoms Associated with PPD*
- Headaches
- Difficulty breathing
- Palpitations
- Fatigue
- Hot flashes/chills
- Panic attacks
- Nausea/upset stomach
- Extreme agitation
- Insomnia
- Excessive sleeping
- Shakiness
- Loss of appetite
- Sugar and/or starch cravings
- Overeating
- Lack of energy
- Poor concentration
- Nightmares

All too often, women believe the uncomfortable and negative feelings they experience have caused their PPD: "I'm so sad and nervous all the time, I must be making myself crazy and depressed!" In fact, the opposite is true—negative feelings are consequences of PPD; they are symptoms.

Look at the following list of emotional symptoms that many women with PPD experience. Some may be familiar to you from different times in your life. Others you may never have experienced before. Don't be alarmed if you find yourself identifying with a great number of them. It is common for most of these feelings to emerge in varying forms at some point during the course of PPD.

Emotional Symptoms Associated with PPD

- Inadequacy
- Poor concentration
- Sadness
- Excessive crying
- Guilt
- Loneliness
- Isolation
- Helplessness
- Anger
- Anxiety
- Resentment
- Fear
- Shame
- Hopelessness
- Loss of control
- Worthlessness
- Lack of confidence
- Irritability
- Thoughts of hurting yourself
- Low self-esteem
- Thoughts of hurting your baby
- Oversensitivity
- Scary thoughts or fantasies
- Confusion
- Feeling "I'm not myself"
- Extreme agitation
- Being overwhelmed
- Inability to laugh
- Depletion

## Scary Feelings

If you are experiencing PPD for the first time, you are probably startled by the range and intensity of emotions you are feeling, as they are often powerful and very frightening. Perhaps the most disturbing are feeling helpless, guilty, suicidal, or angry. If any of your feelings scare you, you should seek professional help immediately.

## "I Can't": Feeling Helpless

Many things become distorted when you are depressed: your moods, your thoughts, your behavior. A negative concept of your immediate world pervades. Jokes aren't funny anymore. Things that you once found pleasurable are barely tolerable now. You're not sure why, but you just don't feel the same way about yourself or things that affect you. Many women start out their sentences with "I can't," indicating what seems like a permanent state of self-doubt and emotional fatigue. They say their greatest fear is that they are going to feel like this forever, that they will never feel confident and positive again.

Feeling helpless is often manifested as a sense of being "stuck," indecisive, or not in charge of your life. Small decisions become major dilemmas, and large decisions can seem insurmountable.

Jane recalls the time she went to the grocery store just after her session with her therapist. She was pleased with her progress and was finally in the mood to treat herself to a nice dinner that she would enjoy making. When she got to the store, she tried to decide what to make. First she thought fish, then she thought veal. She wondered if that would be too expensive, so she thought about chicken. But they had chicken yesterday. So back to fish, but how should she cook it? Was it too cold to barbecue? As she pondered her options, she was amazed at how difficult this task had become. She felt defeated and disappointed.

Feelings of helplessness surface throughout the course of recovery and do not necessarily signal a setback. In general, this is not a good time to make important decisions, since judgment may not be as sharp as usual. Some women find that having a sense of humor about their indecisiveness helps them to cope with the frustration of the moment. Other women, who may be too depressed to find humor in the situation, are better off postponing or delegating decision making for a short time.

## "I'm Letting Everyone Down": Feeling Guilty

In addition to vast pessimism, some of the negative feelings you are now experiencing may be compounded by extreme guilt and shame, which are themselves symptoms of PPD. Sometimes you feel guilt as a result of something you did or didn't do: "I should have stayed home with the baby today instead of going shopping." It can be the result of a feeling you have: "I can't believe it feels so good to be at work, away from the baby"; or it can even be a thought that crosses your mind: "Maybe I should have waited to have this baby." Although many new mothers feel guilty at times, with PPD guilt is almost always more severe and harder to shake off.

While guilt refers to something one did, felt, or thought, shame stretches beyond judging our behavior—it condemns our spirit. Shame refers to how we feel about ourselves deep inside: "If I think that, I must be a terrible person." Shame prevents us from trusting and loving ourselves. It is why it is so difficult to admit that you have any of the negative feelings in the first place: What will people think of me? What kind of person am I?

Mindy was seven months postpartum when she entered therapy.

> I'm so tired of pretending that everything is fine. I'm so tired of crying alone in my room, because I'm afraid of what people would say if they knew how bad I feel. I'm actually embarrassed. I haven't told anyone except my husband. Even my mother thinks I'm just sailing through this. You see, I never did anything right. I'm afraid if I tell them how hard this is for me, they'll say they knew I'd never be able to do this. I just can't admit that I failed again.

Here, we see the immobilizing effect of shame. Mindy sought therapy in an effort to reach out to someone who could listen to her talk about her feelings without judgment and let her know she was okay. The key to overcoming shame is to risk reaching out to someone and talking about whatever is making you feel so badly. It sounds very simple, yet it is very hard to do. Once you can talk about it, you can begin to free yourself of the shame attached to your feelings.

## "I HATE MYSELF. EVERYONE WOULD BE BETTER OFF WITHOUT ME": SUICIDAL THOUGHTS

Lisa was twenty-nine years old when she gave birth to her first baby. She had been depressed for several weeks when she finally consulted a professional for help. Unable to make sense out of her depression on her own, she assumed she was feeling poorly because she wasn't a good mother. She felt very close to her baby, but she cried every time she talked about her. "My baby deserves more than this. She should have a mother who is happy and knows what she is doing. I can't do this," she said through her tears. She put her head down and sighed. "My baby would be better off without me. I don't think I want to die; I just don't want to feel like this anymore. I just want this pain to go away. If I die, would this pain go away?"

Lisa's thoughts of suicide were very passive. Her intent was vague, and she had no plan. But her statements clearly reflect the desperation she felt. Any thoughts of hurting oneself must always be taken seriously. If you are having any thoughts of hurting yourself or are feeling so desperate that you want this sadness to go away at any cost, you must find a professional who can help. Talking about these feelings can help you feel more understood and less alone. Suicidal feelings that are due to PPD are treatable and will resolve with appropriate intervention.

Some women with PPD experience pain that is so intense and so pervasive that they don't want to live. It is critical that you not surrender to these feelings. Reaching out to those who can help you is the single most important thing you can do for yourself right now. Let others know you are feeling this way, and let them take care of you for a change. These thoughts are an indication of a serious depression that can be treated; don't try to deal with them alone. If you are having suicidal thoughts, you need put this book down and call someone right now. For yourself, for your family, for your baby.

## "I'M SICK AND TIRED OF EVERYONE AROUND ME": ANGRY FEELINGS

Another frightening feeling that women with PPD experience is anger at their baby and/or husband. It is difficult to imagine having such animosity toward those closest to you. And when it happens, it doesn't make sense.

- How can I have these horrible feelings toward the baby I love so much?
- Sometimes I just want to scream. I can't stand it if I hear that cry one more time!
- I can't get a minute to myself. I can't eat. I can't wash my hair. I can't even go to the bathroom anymore. I should never have had this baby!
- I just want things to be the way they used to be. I am so tired of this. I don't think I can take anymore. Yesterday when I was making dinner, I spilled juice on the floor and got so mad that I took the container and threw it against the wall. I looked at the mess and felt my body collapse. When I do things like that, it really scares me. What if I hurt my baby?
- My husband can't do anything right. He tries to help me out, but he doesn't have a clue about how I feel. I don't know what makes me think he would understand this!

Anger at your husband or at your baby is one of the most disturbing feelings that women with PPD experience. Most new mothers, including those who do not have PPD, will get angry at their babies from time to time. It is hard to imagine someone not losing her temper after six virtually sleepless nights in a row, or after hearing the baby crying inconsolably for an hour. But it is not easy to express this anger. We live in a culture that doesn't tolerate a mother's rage toward her child even for a moment. We are told: "Don't feel that way," as if a feeling inevitably leads to an action. Therefore, it is understandable that women would deny or block those feelings of anger, almost by instinct.

Think about your own anger. If you are not aware of harboring any, try to think about some of the ways you are responding to different situations. Since anger is so uncomfortable, it is often disguised by more "acceptable" feelings, such as extreme impatience, frustration, or irritability. If you are yelling at your family excessively, exploding in unpredictable outbursts, feeling like every little thing is getting on your nerves, or lashing out in inappropriate situations, consider the possibility that you are misdirecting some anger. When you do not deal effectively with what is really making you angry, it is often expressed impulsively and inappropriately in other areas of your life. If you've been conditioned to be "good" and believe that stifling your anger is one way of keeping it under control, you are wrong. Holding the anger in will eventually cause problems.

### Anger at Your Partner

Sometimes it is hard to tell whether anger is a symptom of PPD or an exacerbation of a preexisting problem. When asked, "Have you ever felt this way toward your husband before?" Marion responded, "Are you kidding? We had a fight on our honeymoon, and we've been fighting ever since!"

On the other hand, women who have rarely felt anger toward their husbands are confused by such unprecedented bitterness. If you are experiencing anger and resentment at your husband, ask yourself these questions: Did I have any of these feelings before the baby was born? Is this a pattern of communication for us? Have I ever felt this way before? If these feelings are brand-new, it is likely that this anger is a symptom of PPD. If you are not sure now, you will know later, when your other symptoms get better. As you recover, if you continue to have anger toward your husband, you will know it is due to an unresolved issue in your basic relationship and not only a symptom of PPD.

### Anger at Your Baby

Being angry at your baby is one of the most terrifying of all emotions. Anger toward your baby can be manifested in feelings of resentment, severe irritation, or exasperation, and may be intermittent or persistent. Although it is a common symptom of PPD, you must take it very seriously. An occasional angry thought toward one's baby is almost universal in mothers with or without PPD. But frequent angry feelings or any angry actions, such as throwing or breaking objects or slapping an older child in an outburst of rage, is very serious.

Many women will harbor these fearful emotions with a secret anguish, hesitant to let anyone know they are so tormented. If you are afraid of these feelings, you are sensing that something is amiss and need to pay attention to your worries and take immediate control. Let others know that you are having these feelings, so they can help you regain perspective. You may need to get someone to help you care for your baby or children until this symptom improves.

It is difficult to think clearly when you are angry, so we have some suggestions to help you at the moment you feel anger toward your baby:

- Isolate yourself from your baby.
- Put your baby in the crib or playpen and let her cry—it is better to let your baby cry than to hit her.
- Go outside if you have to, so you can't hear the crying.
- Take a slow, deep breath. Do this five times.
- Splash your face with cold water.
- If you cannot calm yourself down, call for someone to help you.

The feelings we have discussed in this section are especially painful. In general, the more severe the emotional symptom, the more likely it is that you will need professional help (psychotherapy and/or medication) to manage it. If you are experiencing suicidal thoughts or angry outbursts, we suggest that you proceed to Chapters 6 and 7.

## Emotional Acceptance of PPD

Examine the list of physical sensations and emotional symptoms that we listed previously, and identify those feelings that are most troublesome to you now. List them below, in any order. If you are experiencing a strong feeling that we did not include, add that to your list also. (*Suicidal feelings or feelings that you may hurt your baby do not apply to this exercise. The presence of these feelings warrants immediate intervention.*)

1. _____
2. _____
3. _____
4. _____
5. _____
6. _____
7. _____
8. _____
9. _____
10. _____

So, how do you keep from falling victim to these feelings? Although it may seem paradoxical, the best way to fight these feelings is to let them in—if you don't, the energy you will use trying to hold them back will exhaust you, and ultimately the effort will backfire. Feelings that are resisted take their revenge and can be twice as powerful when they resurface.

Complete the following statements by filling in the blanks with feelings that are most troublesome to you from the list you just wrote. We've all been conditioned to believe that it's not in our best interest to think about negative feelings, but that's not exactly true. What you want to do is confront each feeling you have and give yourself permission to have it for now.

1. I will allow myself to feel

_____

2. I will allow myself to feel

_____

3. I will allow myself to feel

_____

4. I will allow myself to feel

_____

5. I will allow myself to feel

_____

6. I will allow myself to feel

_____

7. I will allow myself to feel

_____

8. I will allow myself to feel

_____

9. I will allow myself to feel

_____

10. I will allow myself to feel

_____

Now, read these statements to yourself. Even if you feel as though you are going through the motions and don't really believe what you are saying to yourself, just repeat the lines. This exercise will help you overcome your fear of these feelings by reducing your resistance to them.

## Owning Your Feelings

Now that you have identified your feelings and can begin to give yourself permission to have them, the next step is to let the feelings in completely by taking responsibility for them. The following points will help make this clear:

- **Accept that these feelings are a very real part of who you are right now:** Even though they feel terrible, remember that they are symptoms of an illness that is very real and very treatable. This is going to get better.

- **Respect your feelings even though they cause such pain:** Just as you would eat if you were hungry or rest if you were tired, you need to take care of yourself when you are experiencing the emotional symptoms of PPD. Reminding yourself that you understand why you feel this way can be very self-nurturing.

- **Don't fight these feelings:** You may think that if you could only stop feeling as you do, you would get over your PPD. Actually, the opposite is true: when your PPD is better, you will stop feeling this way. The emotions you are experiencing are such important symptoms of PPD that we use them as markers in treatment to determine what progress is being made. While you are probably focusing a great deal on how you are feeling right now, you will notice that as your recovery progresses, you will think about your feelings less often. So just take a deep breath and remind yourself that your pain is not going to go away quickly or easily.

- **Don't be afraid of these feelings:** The emotional symptoms of PPD can be unbearable. The pain can seem relentless. But feelings do not automatically lead to actions or behaviors. If you are certain that you will not act on your feelings, try to convince yourself that negative feelings will not make you worse or make the depression last longer. This way, you can begin to break the cycle that is making you continue to feel so badly. (Note: If you continue to experience feelings that are consistently unbearable and frightening to you, it is important that you seek out a professional to help ease this pain.)

## Letting Go: Approaching Total Acceptance

The final stage after you have let each feeling in is to let each one go. This means giving up the hold that these feelings can have over you if you let them; it means understanding that each time you wonder why you are feeling a certain way and try to resist it, you are giving harmful power to that feeling. Letting go means releasing the power a feeling has over you.

It does not mean that you won't feel the pain anymore. It means you will spend less energy questioning your feelings and asking yourself: Why is this happening to me? Why can't I fix this? Why won't this get better? Why am I still feeling this way?

There is nothing terribly sophisticated about the method of letting go. It must simply be allowed to happen on its own as you begin to work through this acceptance process. Try telling yourself that you are just going to feel out of sorts for a while. This is part of who you are right now. Stop ruminating. Stop asking those "why" questions. Stop obsessing. True, this is easier to say than to do. But remind yourself that some of the things you are obsessing about are symptoms, and they will get better. In order to continue to work toward recovery, it is necessary for you to make the transition from "Why is this happening?" to "What can I do about it?"

# ·◦[ 4 ]◦·

# "I'M FALLING APART"

## *Coping Techniques*

*J*UDITH THOUGHT IT WAS GREAT that she had finished all her
thank-you notes. After four months of trying to fit them in, she
finally got the last one out in the mail. But now it was already 11:00
in the morning and her mother-in-law was coming over in a half
hour for lunch. She looked at her house. Toys were all over the place,
breakfast dishes were in the sink, and the casserole dish was dried
out from last night's dinner. She had thirty minutes to get the house
in order. Luckily, the baby was sleeping. Or so she thought, until she
heard her crying upstairs. What was she doing up? She just went
down for her nap a little while ago. Now how would she get everything done? If only she had waited on the thank-you notes—she
would have had time to clean the dishes. Or, if only she had gotten
up a little earlier, or if only she had postponed lunch until next
week, or if only she had . . .

The challenges of everyday life are often overpowering when you have PPD. Sometimes, priorities get all out of whack. Big things slip through the cracks, and little things are blown way out of proportion. There is too much to do, too little time, and too little energy. And there are way too many expectations.

The very first step is to realize that everything will not get done. It is as simple as that. Something has to give. Once you understand this fundamental truth, you will be able to make some choices about what you can let go of, and how to establish healthy expectations for yourself and for others.

## Learning to Set Limits

Setting limits means learning to say no when your instincts, feelings, and body cues are telling you that you are too overwhelmed to say yes. Everyone has difficulty restraining the urge to say yes at one time or another. As women, we are socialized from birth to put others' needs first, and most of us genuinely enjoy the pleasure of caring for someone else.

After the birth of a baby, it is hard to give as much time and energy to family and friends as you once did. When you have PPD, it is impossible to do so. It is absolutely crucial that you begin to establish limits right now that will protect you from anything that may interfere with your effort to take care of yourself in the future. Trying to do the impossible makes you feel depleted, helpless, and even more depressed.

It is particularly hard to erect barriers with people close to you. However, when you are feeling vulnerable, one of the best ways to protect yourself from further intrusions is to create clear and reasonable boundaries. Here are five key elements to help you define and protect your psychic space:

1.  Learn how to distinguish your needs from someone else's and don't back off at the first sign of disagreement.

2. Accept the fact that someone you care about will often not like the limits you set.

3. Admit that you are different right now from how you usually are.

4. Acknowledge that you have needs because you are an individual—not merely someone else's mother, wife, daughter, sister, employee, boss, or neighbor.

5. Recognize the difference between asserting yourself and being selfish or inconsiderate.

## Tolerating Disagreements

Remember Leslie, who had postpartum stress syndrome? A few weeks later, she felt herself on the verge of developing full-blown PPD. Fortunately, she had the strength and confidence to follow her intuition about the best way to avert PPD, even though it meant displeasing her husband by failing to be unconditionally available to their new daughter.

Leslie and her husband agreed that she would take a four-month maternity leave. But, by five-weeks postpartum, Leslie was going stir-crazy. She was lonely and, she had to admit, a little bored with facing the endless parade of dirty dishes and diapers. On impulse, she called her boss, who was delighted when Leslie said she wanted to come to the office two half-days per week for the next three months. Her mother was thrilled to have her granddaughter to herself while Leslie was at work.

That night, Leslie was stunned by her husband's response: "I'm not going to stand in your way, but I don't think it's right for our family. It seems kind of selfish to me to do that to your mom."

Leslie felt a knot in her stomach. Was she being selfish? Was she imposing on her mother? Was it bad for the baby for her to be away for ten hours a week? She burst into tears and left the room. "Fine," she cried. "If that's the way you feel about it, forget the whole thing."

But the next day, she couldn't bring herself to pick up the phone and tell her boss that the new arrangement was off.

That night, Leslie placed a long-distance call to her older sister, who pointed out that this wasn't a situation in which either Leslie or Dan was wrong—they just saw things differently. She encouraged Leslie to do what felt right, pointing out that taking care of her own needs might be best for her and the baby, even if it left Dan feeling uncomfortable. "Dan's a big boy," she said. "He'll deal with it. After all, maybe he's the one being selfish."

Leslie approached Dan again: "I realize that this isn't what we planned, but I also didn't plan to feel so overwhelmed and stressed out. My gut tells me that this is the right decision, and I want to go through with it. If it doesn't help me feel better, or if it seems to be too much for my mother or the baby, we can reconsider. Can you live with that?"

Dan was brusque. "Sure, whatever you want. I said I wouldn't stand in the way." She was disappointed by his half-hearted support, but also glad to have set limits on her compulsion to put everyone else first. It felt great to have something to look forward to that was just for her. Her sister was right—Dan quickly got over it and even seemed excited about the chance to pay off some accumulating bills with the extra money.

## Identifying and Correcting Common Pitfalls

Now take a moment to answer the following questions:

1. Do you have trouble setting limits, especially with loved ones?

   _____

2. In what situations is this most difficult for you?

   _____

3. Do you recall a situation in which you were able to set clear boundaries? If so, how did that feel?

   _____

4. Why do you think it is so hard for you to establish restrictions?

_____

5. What are you afraid will happen if you do?

_____

6. Can you think of some situations that might require you to set limits at this time in your life?

_____

7. Can you begin to identify certain people in your life who need more curbs than others?

_____

8. Can you sort out what makes it so hard to be clear with these people about what you want?

_____

Here are some suggestions for setting limits right now:

- **Set limits on how much you allow the telephone to monopolize your life.** After five minutes, tell callers that you hear the baby crying and need to hang up. Let your phone go straight to voice mail if you don't feel like talking.
- **Restrict visits from family and friends.** Just because someone wants to "come and see the baby" doesn't mean you have to say yes automatically. Consider ways to cut down on visits. For example, instead of having four friends come by separately for visits, ask one to coordinate all five of you getting together somewhere for lunch. Postpone visits—if someone asks to come by on Monday, suggest Thursday. If you are having a bad day, it is okay to reschedule. Tell people, "I'm recovering from childbirth more slowly than I anticipated. Can I call to have you over when I'm feeling stronger?" Most of all, don't succumb to guilt trips hidden in requests to visit: "Is that baby going to be in junior high school before I get to meet him?"

- **Say no when you feel that others are asking too much of you.** One good communication technique for this is to acknowledge that the request is legitimate, but to explain that you simply cannot fulfill it. For example, if your best friend asks to drop her kids by for a few hours while she goes to the doctor, try saying, "I feel terrible that I can't help you out with something so little right now. I just have to say no, even though I know it leaves you stranded. I hope you understand that I'll soon be back to my old self again." Have faith in the friendship—a strong relationship can survive a temporary imbalance in who gives and who takes.

It is important for you to establish and maintain firm limits so you can shield yourself when you're feeling especially vulnerable. Without these limits, you are likely to feel increasingly victimized and less in control. You must trust your instincts about what you need at this time and how best to meet those needs. You cannot go to any length to avoid hurting someone else's feelings, and you are not responsible for making other people happy right now.

## Recognizing Your Stressors

Stress can be defined in terms of economics: demands exceed supply. Demands can be internal or external. The expectations that others place on you, your responsibilities and obligations, and the chores you need to do are all examples of external demands. The wishes and standards that you set for yourself are internal demands. Since taking care of a baby is so all-encompassing, these internal and external demands often accumulate to overwhelm the time, energy, mental concentration, financial resources, and stamina that you have right now. The resulting fatigue, self-doubt, and frustration that you feel are symptoms of stress.

Almost all mothers caring for infants have many more things to do than hours in the day or energy to get them all done. Women with PPD often have a hard time recognizing that a good portion of their stress is typical of caring for a baby and not due to PPD. Since PPD causes guilt and self-criticism, mothers with PPD often feel that everyone else manages the stress better, or that they are incompetent. This self-doubt inhibits them from actively working to reduce stress, and the stress and shame get worse. You need to commit to examining your sources of stress and to work to alleviate them.

Picture yourself as a container that can only hold 100 pennies. If you try to put in 102 or 120 pennies, the container spills over or bursts at the seams. To get back to the amount the container can comfortably hold (the stress you can manage), there are only two options: put less in or take more out. To help you to come up with a stress-reduction plan uniquely tailored to your needs, here are two lists: common postpartum stresses you should minimize (pennies in), and ways to reduce postpartum stress (pennies out).

## COMMON POSTPARTUM STRESSORS

In the course of a typical day, there are a number of things that you do, probably by instinct, that may be contributing to the amount of stress you feel. Although you most likely assume that these chores must get done, and each one may not seem so overwhelming by itself, they can add up to a day filled with tiresome and mundane pressures. Eliminating any or many of these can significantly reduce the overload you will feel on any given day:

- Washing clothes
- Grocery shopping
- Dropping off and picking up dry cleaning
- Making breakfast
- Making dinner
- Entertaining visitors
- Writing thank-you notes for baby gifts
- Packing lunches (for self, partner, kids)

- Vacuuming
- Nighttime feedings
- Doing dishes
- Driving carpool when you have other children
- Pumping breast milk
- Phone calls
- Cleaning the bathroom
- Changing diapers
- Daytime feedings
- Other _____

As you look over the list, notice that these stressors are, of course, made harder by PPD . . . but they are not due to PPD. Many women are surprised to learn that the birth of a first child is considered to be a severe stressor, comparable to divorce. Can you stop criticizing yourself for feeling so burdened? Letting dirty dishes sit in the sink overnight or wearing unlaundered jeans two days in a row doesn't make you an incompetent person—it makes you an ordinary, overloaded mother. The world will not stop turning just because the house is dusty, but you might feel better when you let it go.

## Postpartum Stress Reducers

The list below is designed to help you find ways to reduce these stresses or to balance the stress with self-nurturing. Some common themes emerge: lower your standards on things that aren't top priority, accept imperfection, treat yourself to something special, and obtain a substitute for yourself when possible. We realize that some of these stress reducers may feel like a lighthearted way to combat depression, but research has shown that distraction can prove to be an effective intervention for anxiety. Depression and anxiety can be extremely self-absorbing. We find women feel better when they can divert their attention, even momentarily. Taking extra care of yourself, even by indulging at times, sends the message that you deserve the attention. So while they may or may not make a difference in the bigger picture of your PPD symptoms, we are hoping these suggestions will help you feel a bit better along the way:

- Ask your husband to give the night feedings on the weekend (using formula so you don't have to pump breast milk if you are nursing). This eliminates his "but-I-have-to-be-rested-for-work-tomorrow" issue. Then, let him do it his way and resist the temptation to correct or even make minor suggestions about how the feeding should be done.
- Leave the beds unmade. Close the bedroom door if you don't want any unexpected visitors to see.
- Take a nap while the baby naps. If everyone keeps repeating this advice, isn't it time to try it?
- Take a bath using scented bath oil. Don't wait for a special occasion—do it for yourself. A gentle fragrance sends a subconscious message that you are special and attractive.
- Get hooked on some absurd reality show, and give yourself permission to enjoy it even if it's not realistic, intellectual, or politically correct.
- Have a free makeover done at the cosmetic counter of a department store, just because it feels good to look good. Of course, they will want to sell you their products, so decide in advance what your spending limit is and stick to it. If you can't afford anything, tell them you're so sleep deprived from the new baby that you forgot your wallet/checkbook/cash, so you'll have to come back later.
- Wear sweat pants.
- Take care of your physical self, including exercise and diet (see Chapter 5).
- Simplify dinner. Or order in.

- Simplify your housework. Do the same chores less often or do fewer chores until you feel better. For example, it's okay to change your sheets every other week for a while if you usually do it every week. Likewise, it simplifies things to eliminate certain chores until you're back on your feet.

- Watch a fun movie on TV by yourself during the afternoon.

- Take your baby to a movie that you would enjoy during the day. For the first few months, most infants fall asleep when the noise level goes up. If you arrive at the theater early and feed and change the baby before the movie, you are likely to be able to stay through the entire film. Even if your baby fusses, there probably won't be too many other people there to be disturbed.

- Read a trashy, sizzling romance novel, and really give yourself permission to enjoy it.

- Hire a mother's helper for a couple of hours a day, so you can get a little help while you are also home. Since late afternoon is often the peak time for postpartum stress (right before your husband comes home from work), we recommend having a mother's helper come over right after school (3:00 or 3:30 p.m.). Just having her/him around may allow you to take a better rest, since you won't have to worry about whether you'll wake up if the baby cries. The mother's helper can bring the baby to you for nursing and can burp and change the baby, while you stay in bed. To find a mother's helper, ask a neighbor, someone from church, a friend, or a relative if they know of any kids not yet old enough for solo babysitting. People may guard their babysitters jealously, so please be clear that you are not asking for their sitter. As a side benefit, the mother's helper will be a natural babysitter for you in the future, when she/he is old enough to take that role.

- Ask your mother's helper to wash and dry one or two loads of your baby's laundry.

- Bring your mother's helper with you on errands. For example, taking your baby and your mother's helper along with you will help you get your grocery shopping done more quickly because she/he can carry the baby or give her a bottle while you shop.
- Better yet, treat yourself to an occasional grocery delivery service. You can order groceries online for delivery from many grocery stores.
- Call an old friend you have lost touch with.
- Splurge—have a pizza delivered.
- Go to the mall and treat yourself to a new T-shirt, perfume, or scented candles.
- Get a haircut if you haven't done so since the baby was born. It is okay to be good to yourself.
- Get a manicure or a pedicure or some other superficial treat that helps you feel good.
- Ask your husband to bring home Chinese food.
- If you can, hire a cleaning person or cleaning service, even if it's just once. If you already have a housecleaner, double the frequency of the service on a temporary basis.

## Coping with PPD When You Have Other Children

Having other children when you are suffering from PPD is a major source of stress that deserves special attention. The jealousy toddlers and preschoolers feel toward a new baby is all too common and can easily get on your nerves. To make matters worse, with PPD, your temper flares very easily, and your ability to tolerate sibling rivalry goes way down.

Joan's first postpartum recovery went very well. Sean, now three years old, was an easy baby, the envy of all her friends. The birth of her second child was complicated by an unexpected emergency caesarian and a bout of severe neonatal jaundice. Joan was able to maintain emotional stability, nevertheless, until four weeks postpartum, when a mild case of postpartum depression set in. Joan's biggest problem was Sean: no longer able to command his mother's full attention, he was crushed. Like most three-year-olds, Sean expressed his hurt by acting up: he threw temper tantrums, said "no" just as often as when he was in the terrible twos, and had recently begun repeatedly pinching his new baby sister. He had an uncanny sense of timing, acting his worst when company came or when Joan's mother-in-law was on the phone. Joan was astonished at how her miniature Mr. Hyde turned back into the sweet Dr. Jekyll as soon as her husband came home from work. She found herself snapping at Sean almost constantly, even though she realized that this just made it worse.

There are many excellent books that discuss coping with sibling rivalry, so we won't go into the generalities here. However, we do have some specific suggestions for dealing with sibling rivalry when you have PPD.

- First, take an honest look at whether your anger is out of control. If you are hitting or frequently screaming at your toddler, you should seek professional help to get you through this crisis. One of the indicators of a need for professional treatment is occupational dysfunction, and being out of control as a mother is a form of occupational dysfunction that is every bit as important to recognize as the inability to do any other job.
- Consider whether seeking professional advice for your child might help him overcome his sibling rivalry.
- Use distractions to break the cycle of escalating tempers. Get about ten ultra-cheap toys and wrap them in old comics. When the baby is hungry and crying and your preschooler is choosing that very minute to reach new levels

of whining, grab a "big brother" present from your reserves and use it. Say, "This is for you to play with until we have a chance to be together." As soon as you can, cuddle together and let him know how much you love him. Of course, bribery is not a long-term child-rearing method. Think of this as something that helps you get through the small crises of the postpartum transition when you have PPD. You will not spoil your child if you use this technique sparingly for a few weeks. Turning on a children's movie can also be helpful for deescalating tensions.

⚜ Tell your child about PPD in terms he can understand. Expect that he has noticed and is scared or concerned, even if he hasn't said anything. Try: "Mommy doesn't feel good right now. Sometimes this happens to mommies after having a new baby. The sickness makes Mommy cry sometimes and makes Mommy get mad a lot. It's not because of anything you did or because we don't love each other enough. Just like you sometimes get sick and then get better, I will be better again, too. No matter how sick I feel, I always know how much I love you."

⚜ Avoid harsh words as much as possible. Remember that your child's self-esteem is especially vulnerable right now. Children normally view themselves as the center of the universe and the cause of all that happens. Your child may feel responsible for your illness and may feel that you are mad at him because he is making you sad. Remind him that this is not so.

⚜ Call in reserve caretakers as much as possible.

## Passing Time

With PPD, time becomes distorted in one of two ways. In mild cases, time flies by, even though it never feels productive. There aren't enough hours in the day to get everything you planned done, and it seems that everything takes longer than it should. Other sections of this book, on stress reduction, setting limits, changing expectations, and taking care of your physical self, are geared to those who can't find the time they wish they had.

In severe cases or during periods of severe flare-ups, time is insufferably slowed down. Each minute is a torture to be endured. Women who are taking antidepressant medication or are hospitalized for the severest forms of PPD experience time as going by extremely slowly. In an inpatient treatment ward, time is very structured, with therapeutic activities planned throughout the day. While the majority of women with PPD are able to function well enough to remain at home, many find themselves waiting for each minute to pass. There is no easy answer for this, but we have a few suggestions that might help.

Time is very slow if you are in a state of agitation, in which every second drags by. You probably know whether this applies to you—if you have times when you feel like you want to crawl out of your skin, this is common with high levels of agitation. Relaxation techniques are particularly useful, because they combat agitation by helping you regain focus when your thoughts are jumping and spinning around. They may help you calm down enough to fall asleep, which is a good way to pass time. Even if you don't sleep, relaxation techniques break time up into smaller segments, which pass more quickly. Anyone with any form of PPD can try these relaxation techniques—you don't have to be in a state of panic to feel refreshed from a relaxation exercise.

- Listen to a relaxation or mindfulness audio CD. Some people prefer sounds of ocean waves or a waterfall, or of course, your favorite music. Or, have someone record the following visualization exercise for you (this should be read in a calm, very slow manner).

- Close your eyes and take a few slow, deep breaths. Now picture yourself on a beach. . . . Feel the warm sun on your skin. . . . Listen to the sound of the ocean as the waves roll in . . . and roll out. . . . Hear the seagulls. . . . Feel the warm sand underneath your towel. . . . Smell the scents of the beach, the saltwater, and the suntan lotion. . . . Continue to take several slow, deep breaths as you feel your body let the tension flow out.
- Take the baby out in a stroller or carrier/sling and go for a walk around your neighborhood.
- Drink warm milk or herbal tea.
- Take a hot bath.
- Ask your husband to rub lotion or baby powder on you, or get a professional therapeutic massage (from a licensed masseuse only).
- Find some good comedies or light dramas to watch, especially during the day.

## THE POWER OF PLAY

Sometimes, in the course of growing up, our adult selves inhibit us from taking care of ourselves as well as we did as children. Remember how good it felt to get really messy without an inner voice telling you not to dirty the floor? Remember how good it felt to make a lot of loud, uncensored noise? Remember how good it felt to lie down on top of that big hill outside and roll down, without worrying that you might get grass stains all over your clothes? Remember how good it felt to run and play in the rain when there was no adult around to tell you to come inside before you catch pneumonia?

All of these memories tap into an earlier time, when you were unburdened by the resistances and constraints acquired during the transition to adulthood. Play means different things to different people. Try to recall elements of earlier forms of play that would feel heavenly to you now. If you are really good at this, you will choose some playful ideas that make you feel a little bit silly, a little bit embarrassed, and maybe even a little bit guilty! For example, have you ever tried making yourself laugh aloud? It's good for you. Or, how about dancing to an old song, or singing loudly along with your car radio? Some other guilty pleasures might be: watching reality shows on television, playing computer games, enjoying an old soap opera from days past, or checking out videos of cute baby animals on YouTube. All of these distractions have the potential to relax your brain and soothe your weary soul.

*Do not underestimate the power that rediscovering play can have in your life.* Do something outrageous. Or do something ridiculous. Or do something that's plain old fun.

And if this is too much for you to do right now, just remember this idea and use it later. When you are feeling better, play can open many windows that facilitate better relaxation, communication, sexuality, and intimacy.

## REGAINING CONTROL

Every new mother, and especially those with PPD, will experience loss of control, to some extent, in some area of her life. Not all women with PPD will choose or will need to seek professional assistance to get their lives back on track. In this chapter, we have suggested specific self-help techniques that will help you regain some of this control. How you feel at any given time will determine what you decide to do about it. For example, if you are feeling so overwhelmed that it is difficult for you to get out of bed in the morning, then treating yourself to a manicure is clearly not the appropriate action to take. If, on the other hand, you are feeling tired because you've been running around with the kids all day and haven't had a minute to yourself, then the idea of a nice, warm bubble bath may sound like heaven and will be a wonderful short-term solution.

# Crisis Management

"Coping" involves adapting to stress. Your ability to cope is directly affected by the nature of your case of PPD, which is not under your control. If you have a milder version of the illness, you may be able to implement a few ideas about coping and make significant improvement. However, if you have a severe form, coping may require you to take aggressive—and sometimes scary—steps, including professional treatment or even hospitalization. If so, keep in mind that your prognosis is still quite good—with appropriate intervention, it will eventually be much easier to cope.

This part of the chapter is for women who are in profound distress. When PPD is at its most severe, coping literally means getting through each day, a day at a time.

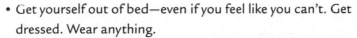

### HOW DO I GET THROUGH THE DAY?

- Get yourself out of bed—even if you feel like you can't. Get dressed. Wear anything.
- Brush your teeth. Wash your face. Brush your hair.
- Leave your bed unmade.
- Tell yourself it is okay to get away with doing only the very minimum today. The only things that MUST be done are: All children must be dressed, fed, changed, held, napped, fed again, etc. IF YOU DO NOT FEEL CAPABLE OF TAKING CARE OF YOUR BABY'S AND/OR OTHER CHILDREN'S BASIC NEEDS, IT IS IMPERATIVE THAT YOU CALL SOMEONE TO HELP YOU CARE FOR THEM.
- Allow yourself some time to cry. Curl up on the couch, and after you have cried for ten minutes, take a deep breath and get up.

*—continues—*

*—continued—*

- Make a list of a couple of things you might be able to handle today. These things will vary from day to day, depending on how you feel. For example: call a friend, read a magazine, take a walk, invite someone over, write in a journal, go shopping, watch TV.
- You don't have to do the laundry today. You don't have to clean the kitchen floor today. It may make you feel better if you put the dishes in the dishwasher. Set very small goals for yourself. Remember, one step at a time.
- You don't have to make dinner today. Have your husband bring home takeout, or order food delivered.
- Try not to watch the clock. ("It's only 10:30 in the morning—how am I going to make it through the rest of the day?") If you find that you can't stop watching the clock, then find a funny picture, or a cartoon, or print a large list of thoughts that make you feel good and post one of these right next to the clock so that it distracts you.
- You can cry again. Remember to give yourself ten minutes.
- Find yourself a special stuffed animal, one that belongs only to you, either an old one that has particular sentimental value or a special new one from the store. Keep this stuffed animal with you when you are home. Give it a name. Hug it. Hold it when you cry. It can help you feel safe and loved, if you let it.
- Call your husband and let him know how you are doing. Don't wait for him to call you. If you have to call him three times a day, that's okay for now. Let him know you appreciate his support.
- Remember to ask for help if you need it.

If even getting through the day is too much, you need to consider a partial hospitalization program or inpatient hospitalization. A partial program (also known as an IOP, Intensive Outpatient Program) is a day-treatment program that concentrates on group therapy and individual psychiatric attention. You would attend daily programs and return home in the evening. Women who need more intense structure, or whose symptoms disable them from functioning may benefit from inpatient hospitalization. Although this may be very frightening, if it will ease your distress and speed your recovery, it is an option well worth considering.

If you or your doctor and/or therapist feel that being in the hospital would be in your best interest right now, we hope that you will consider the possibility that this will actually make things better, even though it may be very scary. Intensive treatment and relief from all the pressures of home may be just what you need to get back on track. Many women with PPD are afraid that they will be "locked up" forever. Fortunately, even when hospitalization for PPD is necessary, the prognosis for full recovery is excellent.

---

### I CAN'T COPE—SHOULD I GO TO THE HOSPITAL?

Hospitalization is usually necessary when:

- You are suicidal.
- You are psychotic (hearing voices, feeling paranoid, or having delusional beliefs).
- There is actual risk of harm to the baby.
- You are unable to perform the necessary basics of daily activities, such as eating, dressing, or getting out of bed.

*—continues—*

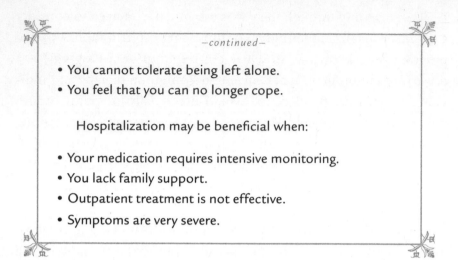

*—continued—*

- You cannot tolerate being left alone.
- You feel that you can no longer cope.

  Hospitalization may be beneficial when:

- Your medication requires intensive monitoring.
- You lack family support.
- Outpatient treatment is not effective.
- Symptoms are very severe.

# ·[ 5 ]·

# "I'm Tired, Fat, Ugly, and Still Wearing My Nightgown at Noon"

## Making Time to Take Care of Yourself

*Nobody would believe what an effort it is to do what little I am able.*
—CHARLOTTE PERKINS GILMAN, *THE YELLOW WALLPAPER*, 1892

FINDING TIME TO CARE FOR HERSELF is one of the most important yet most difficult challenges for a woman with PPD. For many women, the effort it takes to do what the baby, the house, other children, and/or the job require leaves no leftover energy for self-nurturing. For others, it just doesn't feel right to put one's own needs first. But neglecting yourself is costly; eventually, you become so worn down that you are unable to nurture anyone else.

We feel very strongly that when you have PPD, taking care of your physical self is a necessity, not a luxury that you can put on hold. There is a direct connection between how well you eat, sleep, rest, and exercise, and how you feel emotionally. It is imperative that you pay attention to the signals your body sends out and learn how to take care of yourself, little by little.

Below are some typical statements made by women in the first few postpartum weeks. Check any that describe your situation.

_____ 1.  I can't stand any of my clothes. My pre-pregnancy outfits are too tight, and it's just too humiliating to wear my maternity clothes.

_____ 2.  I know that everyone says I should sleep when the baby does, but I just can't. There's too much to do during her nap.

_____ 3.  I know that I would feel better if I started exercising again. But who has time to go to the gym?

_____ 4.  Grabbing a candy bar on my way home from work gives me the strength I need to face those first few minutes when I walk in the door and my four-year-old starts whining, and the dog needs to be let out, and the baby wants to be nursed.

_____ 5.  Give up caffeine? No way. I can't. Never. No.

_____ 6.  Why bother taking a shower? There's no one here to see me anyway.

Did we catch you neglecting your physical self? Don't feel embarrassed—almost all new mothers have to struggle with these pitfalls. Because physical health is crucial for emotional well-being, we are going to discuss basics about sleep, exercise, self-care, and nutrition in this chapter.

## Exercise

Jennifer was a flight attendant before she married Bill. She never considered herself to be gorgeous, not like some of the women she worked with, but she knew that her careful dieting and regular aerobics classes paid off in a great figure. Jennifer and Bill were in their early thirties when they married, and both were anxious to start a family right away. Jennifer got pregnant six months after they married.

Her first trimester was awful—she had severe morning sickness and fatigue and couldn't find the energy to work out anymore. She ate crackers constantly to ward off the nausea, and shocked herself by gaining eleven pounds in the first three months, despite eating barely anything but crackers. In later months, she couldn't resist her cravings for ice cream and donuts. She was tired all the time and never got back into the routine of her spin class. By the time her daughter was born, Jennifer had gained forty-two pounds.

For almost two weeks after the baby was born, Jennifer still looked pregnant, and a few strangers even asked her when her baby was due. She couldn't fit into any of her old clothes and wore her bathrobe most days just to avoid putting on her maternity clothes. She felt guilty about her looks, certain that Bill regretted a) ever meeting her, b) marrying her, and c) having a baby with her. Since she was nursing, her appetite remained robust, and besides, eating something high in calories was the only temporary relief she ever got from the demands of the day. But she felt worse each time she looked in the mirror. She hated her stretch marks and tried to cover them up whenever Bill caught a glimpse of her showering. She couldn't seem to stop thinking about the beautiful women Bill encountered at work each day and hated herself for becoming what she thought was a stereotypical fat, jealous housewife.

Jennifer's feelings of being unattractive are related to having postpartum stress syndrome. She's overwhelmed and doesn't know how to make her own needs a priority. She is caught in a vicious cycle—she believes that exercise is impossible and sees eating as the only pleasurable activity of the day. She is using food to nurture herself, as a familiar friend during moments of despair. Not being able to lose the weight she put on during pregnancy perpetuates her low self-esteem, which perpetuates a feeling of being out of control, which paralyzes her and makes her turn to food. Bill did just the right thing:

> One Sunday afternoon, Bill offered to go with Jennifer to their gym and to take care of the baby while she worked out. It felt so good! Jennifer hadn't realized how important exercise was for her, both physically and mentally. At her six-week checkup, her doctor had okayed exercise as long as it wasn't painful or for more than an hour a day. Jennifer called around and found a mother-baby exercise class that met twice a week. After three weeks, she realized that exercise had gone from being torture to being a treat that she craved. She found that her old gym didn't mind her bringing the baby to class with her, and she got back to her routine of working out four or five days a week. She noticed that other women in the locker room had stretch marks, too, and no one felt like the ugliest woman in America. Since she couldn't wear her bathrobe to exercise class, she bought some large stretch pants and an oversized shirt that Bill told her was the most beautiful outfit she ever owned! She found that exercise helped her feel more in control of her body, and she was able to reassert the power that she had seemed to lose to pregnancy, cravings, childbirth, and stretch marks.

This book is filled with advice, some of which will feel right to you and that you will try, and some of which you will reject immediately as "not for me." Please give this piece of advice a try, even if it seems "not for me." Whether you have been a couch potato all your life or an exercise maniac, postpartum exercise can be extremely beneficial. Many people report an antidepressant effect from exercise, which is believed to release brain chemicals called endorphins that evoke a feeling of well-being. One recent study found that people who were very inactive were almost twice as likely as those who were physically active to become depressed. Although this study did not address PPD specifically, we often see the tremendously beneficial effect of exercise in our practices.

Exercise is also beneficial for postpartum anxiety and panic. Consistent aerobic exercise alters body metabolism and will help you avoid sudden buildups of lactic acid, a substance that induces panic attacks. Many women with panic disorder are greatly helped by exercise.

Here are some tips on postpartum exercise:

- Always check with your obstetrician or midwife for medical clearance. This is especially important if you have had a caesarian, are fewer than six weeks postpartum, have not recently been exercising, or have any preexisting medical illness. But remember, check with your doctor even if you don't have any of these special circumstances.

- Sign up for a mother-baby class. There are all sorts of classes, including music, gym, and yoga, with babies of all ages. Since many women with PPD believe that they are the only one having "bad mother" feelings, being around lots of other postpartum women will help you sort out what is normal postpartum stress and what is PPD. It can be eye opening to see a "regular" mother get angry when her baby wakes up five minutes into the workout or to overhear someone complaining about how it took her two hours just to get out of the house to come to class. If loneliness is a problem right now, ask one of the class members to go for coffee after class.

- If nursing, be sure to wear a very supportive bra.

- Avoid high-impact exercises—take a low-impact class, or use equipment such as a treadmill or stationary bike for your workout.

- If your facility has a whirlpool, use it after class for relaxation—set the baby in his/her infant seat at the side. (This won't work if your baby is crawling or walking.)

- Don't overlook a vigorous walk as excellent postpartum exercise, free-of-charge. Studies have proven that brisk walking has physiological benefits comparable to other types of aerobic exercise. Walk at about the pace you would if you were almost late to an appointment. You can't really walk for aerobic exercise pushing a stroller and stopping at every curb, so you may want to bring the stroller to an outdoor track or to a walking trail at a park. Try using an infant carrier (or a backpack if your baby is older) if your pediatrician approves. Otherwise, go for a twenty-minute walk before your husband leaves for work or after he comes home. Sometimes, it works best for all three of you to go out: Dad carries the baby, and you both walk briskly. Aim for doing this three times a week.

- If you suffer from panic attacks, be sure to build up your exercise tolerance at a gradual pace. If you do too much too quickly, you will have a sudden surge in lactic acid, a natural metabolite released when your muscles are not conditioned. Lactic acid has been shown to cause panic attacks in a laboratory setting. Aerobic exercise actually changes how your muscles use oxygen—when done gradually, aerobic exercise will minimize how much lactic acid your body releases.

## Eating Right

Poor nutrition is extremely common in women with PPD. One of two patterns is usually seen: 1) sugar and carbohydrate cravings, increased appetite, diminished willpower, and attempts to self-medicate with high-calorie food ("I feel so bad that I am going to relieve my suffering for a few moments with this chocolate"); or 2) total lack of appetite, food all tastes the same (bad), and overly rapid weight loss.

While both patterns represent symptoms of PPD, the poor nutrition that results can make PPD worse, both directly and indirectly. Inadequate nutrition can cause vitamin deficiencies and contribute to fatigue. Eating poorly can further lower fragile self-esteem when you criticize yourself for doing what you know you shouldn't. Right now, it is very important that you keep your physical health up. Following are a few ideas for healthier ways to eat, pitfalls to avoid, and practical suggestions. Consider a comprehensive evaluation by a dietician or nutritionist (your doctor should be able to recommend one), especially if you are breastfeeding or have a noticeable change in your dietary habits or weight.

## Nutritional Pitfalls in PPD

We realize that the easiest way to eat right now is to grab the first thing at hand that doesn't require any preparation. Potato chips, ice cream bars, and a soda are easiest. Making salads, peeling carrots, and cutting grapefruit seem like too much effort. Junk food can actually aggravate your distress, however, so we recommend that you avoid all of the following:

- Anything with caffeine: coffee, tea, colas, other caffeinated soft drinks, chocolate. Except for chocolate, these substances all come in decaffeinated versions. Check soft drink labels carefully, because many contain caffeine when you wouldn't expect them to. Likewise, "herbal" teas may contain caffeine, so read the fine print. Caffeine is a central nervous system stimulant that may trigger anxiety attacks and contribute to insomnia, making PPD worse. Since all parents of infants are chronically exhausted, it is very tempting to consume lots of caffeine. We recommend total abstinence. If you currently consume a lot of caffeine-containing beverages, wean yourself gradually to avoid caffeine-withdrawal headaches. Try cutting back your consumption by 50 percent every two days.

⚬ Concentrated carbohydrates: candy, cakes, donuts, ice cream, and sugary beverages, including regular soft drinks and sugar-containing powdered beverage drinks. These cause rapid swings in your blood sugar that can mimic or trigger panic attacks. Panic attacks are often due to misinterpretation of normal physiological changes, such as normal increases in heart rate. Someone who is oversensitized to her body's signals may experience this as an anxiety attack, when in fact it is due to normal, benign physiological adjustments. It may be very helpful to avoid these rapid sugar highs and lows.

⚬ Fried and high-fat foods: substitute a taco salad for a cheeseburger at the local fast-food joint.

⚬ Alcohol: alcohol is a brain depressant that also causes sleep disruption. Whether the alcohol is in the form of beer, wine, hard liquor, or mixed beverages doesn't matter. Many well-intentioned people (sometimes even doctors) will advise a mother with PPD to "have a glass or two of wine at bedtime," or "have a beer to keep your milk supply up."

There are two common old wives' tales about alcohol that are not correct. The first is that alcohol is good for breastfeeding mothers or for promoting milk supply or milk letdown. It's been shown that babies whose mother took only one alcoholic beverage nursed less well and gained less weight than babies whose mothers had none. Breast milk transmits alcohol from mother to baby; since you would never add alcohol to a baby's bottle, don't add it to your breast milk, even if someone tells you that it's good for stress relief.

The second misconception is that alcohol promotes sleep. While alcohol does tend to induce sleep at first, a few hours later it promotes what is called "middle insomnia." Alcohol will make you wake up a few hours after falling asleep and then keep you up for the rest of the night.

Most importantly, regular alcohol consumption will directly cause a depressed mood. Stay away from it for now.

## HEALTHIER EATING HABITS WHEN YOU HAVE PPD

Along with the nutritional "don'ts," there are also important nutritional "do's." Many of you learned good nutrition in your childbirth-preparation classes. The advice you received there applies to this illness as well. Many of us know what we should do nutritionally—we just don't make it a priority or we fall into bad habits. Following are positive ways you can improve your nutrition as part of recovering from postpartum depression and anxiety. These are realistic and can be done even when you are feeling your worst.

- Increase the amount of complex carbohydrates in your diet. These include whole-grain breads, whole-grain cereals such as bran flakes or oatmeal, grains such as kasha or bulgur wheat, potatoes (not fried), rice, and whole-grain pasta. While we used to believe that all carbohydrates were too fattening, we now know that excess fat (butter, shortening, oil) is the real culprit. Complex carbohydrates help keep your blood-sugar level steady without the big ups and downs that sugary foods cause. Stay away from heavily refined or processed carbohydrates.
- Try to eat smaller, more frequent meals. One woman we treated described anxiety attacks every evening. When we realized that she was putting off dinner until her husband came home (8:00 or 9:00 p.m.), we recommended a 5:00 p.m. snack. She decided to combine two bits of dietary advice and added a 5:00 p.m. bowl of oat bran to her routine. It made a big difference. Your body will interpret hunger as anxiety, which can trigger panic attacks.

- Increase your intake of fresh fruits and vegetables.
- If you have sugar cravings and weight gain, substitute "light" products. For example, substitute fat-free or sugar-free frozen yogurt for regular ice cream. Try sugar-free decaffeinated soft drinks or sugarless beverages such as water with a slice of lemon, flavored seltzer, or plain herbal iced tea.
- Talk to your doctor or midwife about continuing your prenatal vitamins until you are over the PPD. Although it is extremely rare, a vitamin deficiency can mimic PPD. However, megavitamins can be dangerous, so avoid the extremes.
- If you absolutely have to have that slice of cheesecake, have it at the end of a meal rather than as a snack by itself. This protects you from big fluctuations in blood sugar.
- Buy prepared vegetables at the market. Surrender to the premade salad mixes with lettuce already washed and torn, cut-up carrot sticks, celery sticks, broccoli, and cauliflower. Yes, they're ridiculously expensive, but this is only a temporary expenditure to help you get through this rough period.
- Fresh fruits are perfect for snacking. Bananas require absolutely no preparation and are just as easily eaten as a cupcake. Apples and grapes only require washing—bring a few apples with you to snack on at work, or leave a few out on the kitchen counter each day.
- Low-fat yogurt is another healthy food that requires no preparation. You can pack it for lunch at work or eat it at home with no effort.
- Substitute a frozen light dinner for take-out fast food (examples include: Lean Cuisine, SmartOnes, Healthy Choice, Kashi frozen entrees, etc.). The cost is about the same, but the food is a bit better for you.
- Don't grocery shop on an empty stomach. Hunger will make you much more likely to pick up the high-sugar goodies that will only tempt you once they are in your cupboard.

## FOR THOSE WITH NO APPETITE

Try either of these as often as you can—up to five or six times per day if you aren't eating regular foods.

1. Ask your pharmacist or doctor to recommend a nutritional supplement such as Ensure or Sustacal. These are flavored liquid high-protein, high-calorie supplements that help you keep up your strength when you have no appetite. Many women with PPD-related loss of appetite find it easier to take in liquids rather than solids.

2. Add powdered milk, wheat germ, and some frozen orange juice concentrate or honey to a yogurt-based fruit smoothie for extra nutritional power. Example: in a blender puree 1 cup of fresh berries, 1 cup vanilla yogurt, 1 tablespoon wheat germ, 1–2 tablespoons of thawed frozen orange juice concentrate, and 3 or 4 ice cubes.

## LOSING THAT POSTPARTUM WEIGHT

Crash diets (liquid diets, all-juice diets, cleanses, severe calorie-restriction diets) are not a good idea right now. We all know of new mothers who walked out of the hospital wearing the same size-4 jeans they  wore before they were pregnant, but these women are the exceptions. The majority feel overweight, have lost abdominal muscle tone, and generally don't care much for their postpartum bodies. Try hard to accept yourself as you are. There is plenty of time to get back in shape. Be reasonable about your weight-loss goals—being at your pre-pregnancy weight by your child's first birthday is much more reasonable than aiming for that by the end of the first month. Sensible weight-loss plans include careful dietary planning and exercise, not self-starvation.

## WHEN YOU STILL HAVE YOUR NIGHTGOWN ON AT NOON

We understand how difficult it is to take care of your appearance right now. With all that you have to do and with very little energy to do it, you don't have much time for yourself. The poor self-image that is part of PPD often includes a poor body image. It also causes a sense of hopelessness—you may feel so ugly that you begin to feel you are a lost cause. This can lead to a vicious cycle—not bothering with your appearance can lead to even lower self-esteem, which per-petuates PPD.

We include taking care of your physical appearance here, because attending to your physical health is a package that includes eating right, exercising, resting enough, and caring about the basics of your appearance. Letting one area go has a domino effect on the other ar-eas: if you haven't had a haircut for four months, you probably aren't tending to other physical needs either. If you feel like an ugly blob, you won't find the strength to make eating right a priority.

Here are a few suggestions for making yourself feel more attrac-tive during the postpartum period. We estimate these will not take you more than ten minutes each to accomplish. See what you can manage.

- Get dressed, even if you can't get to it until 10:00 a.m. or so. Wearing your nightgown all day is definitely the easiest route, but no one looks or feels fit or pretty in anything worn day after day.
- Put on a little makeup, even if you won't see anyone else all day. You deserve to look pretty, just for yourself. If you really don't have the energy, just apply mascara. Maybe add lipstick or lip gloss. You give yourself a subliminal message every time you pass a mirror when you do this: "My ap-pearance matters."

⚬ If you're like Jennifer, and you gained a lot of weight during pregnancy, don't only wear old maternity clothes. Buy yourself at least two outfits that fit now, even though you know you'll be too thin for them in no time. Consider these an extension of your maternity wardrobe, another expense of having a baby. You can always find things at discount outlets or Marshalls or TJ Maxx. Alternatively, buy items that can adapt to your anticipated slimmer body (such as leggings) or that can be easily altered. After you lose weight, pack them away with your maternity clothes, if you're considering having another baby, or give them to a homeless women's shelter in your area.

## BEWARE OF THE PERFECTION TRAP

Once in a while, women with acute PPD show up at our offices looking like they stepped out of a *Vogue* advertisement. They manage to look great on the outside, but we often wonder at what cost. If this sounds like you, consider the possibility of easing up a little. This might include cutting back on the time you spend on makeup, or wearing jeans more often. For new mothers, perfection is a very tough standard to meet. Perfectionism often masks deep feelings of shame and insecurity. It's a trap, though, because it prevents you from actively working on self-acceptance, and it squanders precious energy.

# Postpartum Depression and Insomnia

The vast majority of women with PPD suffer from chronic sleep deprivation, chronic insomnia, and severe fatigue. As we mentioned in the first chapter, sleep disturbances cause some forms of PPD. In other cases, sleep disturbances are symptoms of PPD.

Sleep deprivation in the first few postpartum weeks is almost universal, since new babies almost never sleep through the night.

Repeated interrupted sleep precipitates or aggravates certain types of PPD, most commonly anxiety and less commonly postpartum psychosis. In other cases, sleeplessness is the first symptom of PPD, with mood changes following the sleeplessness. Difficulty falling asleep or staying asleep, even when the baby sleeps, is a classic symptom of PPD. There are several types of insomnia patterns seen in PPD. Which best describes you?

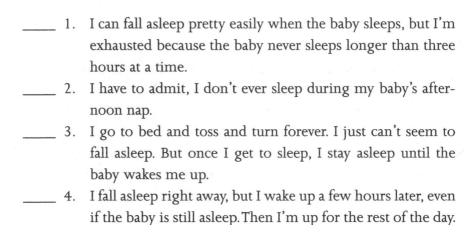

_____  1.  I can fall asleep pretty easily when the baby sleeps, but I'm exhausted because the baby never sleeps longer than three hours at a time.

_____  2.  I have to admit, I don't ever sleep during my baby's afternoon nap.

_____  3.  I go to bed and toss and turn forever. I just can't seem to fall asleep. But once I get to sleep, I stay asleep until the baby wakes me up.

_____  4.  I fall asleep right away, but I wake up a few hours later, even if the baby is still asleep. Then I'm up for the rest of the day.

The first two statements are commonly seen in postpartum stress syndrome. The third statement describes a condition called "initial insomnia." It is especially common in postpartum anxiety syndromes. The fourth statement is called "late insomnia" or "early-morning wakening." This is quite common in "typical" postpartum depression. The rest of this chapter focuses on these patterns individually. It is possible to have two types (for example, stress and anxiety insomnia), so be sure to look over all of the sections that apply to you. (Remember: these are just generalizations. You may have none of these patterns and still have PPD.)

## POSTPARTUM STRESS SLEEP DEPRIVATION: UNAVOIDABLE?

Women with postpartum stress syndrome are often perfectionists who feel guilty if they "waste time" sleeping when they could be doing something else. Even worse is the guilt they feel if they fail to provide instantaneous mom/bottle/breast/cuddle at any and all times, day and night. When you feel like a failure, it's hard to see depriving your baby of even a few minutes of instant gratification as a positive step. For this reason, we spend a lot of time in our practices encouraging stressed-out mothers to set some limits on the tyranny of sleepless nights.

Some sleep deprivation is unavoidable. It is a very rare baby who sleeps through the night right away. The nervous system (including the part of the brain that regulates sleep) continues to develop after birth. Until their nervous systems mature, newborns generally lack the ability to sleep for long stretches. This usually happens somewhere in the range of four or five months of age, although it varies from infant to infant.

Once babies reach four or five months, they generally have less of a biologic need to wake you up. It's mostly social at this point—they enjoy the middle-of-the-night visit with you. Babies sleep in short two-to-four-hour cycles (unlike adults, whose cycle averages eight hours). All babies wake up in the middle of the night—the baby who "sleeps through the night" is actually a baby who puts himself back to sleep after he wakes up. Since your baby is waking up at 1:00 or 2:00 a.m., from his point of view, it makes perfect sense to get you up, too. What could be more fun?

In general, older babies can be taught to get themselves back to sleep. The hard part when you have PPD is holding back from immediately soothing a crying baby. Some mothers feel so insecure, that they have mixed feelings about giving up the small amount of self-affirmation that a nighttime cuddle provides.

Although we encourage you to work with your older baby to help him sleep through the night (with the approval of your pediatrician or family doctor), *do not do this if it makes you feel worse*. If the suggestions below increase your worry or cause you more self-doubt, do not continue this effort. These are simply ideas that may help those mothers who feel ready to work on their infant's sleep patterns. If successful, this may help your PPD, because a stretch of six or seven hours of uninterrupted sleep can be a major part of your recovery. We suggest that you talk this over with your baby's doctor—pediatricians and family doctors who treat babies are experts in this area and can tell you whether your baby is ready. We have also listed some books on this subject in the Recommended Reading section at the end of the book.

The first part of encouraging your baby to sleep through the night is to recognize that how your baby sleeps does not reflect on *you.* Strangers, relatives, physicians, colleagues at work, and even repairmen feel free to comment on your baby's sleep patterns and often seem to be judging you by the duration of your infant's sleep. Sleep is not evidence of anything to do with your mothering skills. It is a natural process that will regulate itself regardless of what you do or don't do.

The following are tips that we have used for our own babies and that we find most women with PPD can manage.

- After your baby is two weeks old, try to avoid letting her sleep longer than three hours at a time during the day. Wake her up after three hours for a feeding. Keep her near the hustle and bustle during the day to try to help her wake up on her own.

- After your baby is four weeks old, try not to let her sleep longer than two hours at a time during the day. Wake her up after two hours for a feeding. We realize that it can feel almost masochistic to wake up a sleeping infant when you may have just finally sat down for a few minutes, but it pays off later.

- After your baby reaches four or five months of age, try to avoid going to her immediately when she starts to wake after her first three-to four-hour sleep cycle. Do this by giving her a few minutes before you jump to the rescue. This takes discipline, because thirty seconds of listening to your baby crying can feel like a year. Watch the clock, and let five minutes go by before you pick her up. If five minutes seems impossible, try three at first and work up to five. Later, try seven or eight. If after whatever period of time you feel comfortable waiting your baby is still crying, try to soothe her with a pacifier, a pat or rub, and your voice. Nurse or give her a bottle only when all else fails.

* By four months, begin laying your baby down to sleep at night while she is still awake. This teaches her to fall asleep in her crib while awake. That way, when she wakes up in the middle of the night, she already knows how to fall asleep by herself in her own crib. A baby who is only put into her crib after she falls asleep may panic upon awakening after her four-hour sleep cycle, because she doesn't know how to fall asleep when not held, rocked, nursed, sung to, and so on.

* Occasionally, babies who have taught themselves to sleep through the night get out of the habit if they are teething or have a fever after an immunization, or if an ear infection has interrupted nighttime sleep. Obviously, a baby who wakes up in pain should be comforted immediately. But once you are certain that the source of the pain has resolved, try to stretch out the time interval before you enter her room or pick her up. For example, at first wait five minutes before going in (if you can). After calming her down, leave and wait ten minutes. Then go back in, calm her down, and let her cry another fifteen minutes. A few nights of this should get her back in her routine. If this is too hard for you, please don't make yourself feel worse by trying to do the impossible.

## POSTPARTUM STRESS AND NAPS

We cannot overemphasize the importance of taking a rest during your baby's nap. Do not do the laundry, cook dinner, mop the floor, write thank-you notes, address birth announcements, or otherwise lift a finger during your baby's nap.

Of course, if this were so easy you would have already done it, right? Trust us, this is the single most important piece of advice we can give you.

# Letting Go

What is getting in the way of your rest? How can you let go?

Is it *perfectionism*? Do you write thank-you notes during your baby's nap because you tell yourself: "If I don't, people will think I am rude"? If so, try letting go by accepting being good enough. Tell yourself: "Late thank-you notes for a new-baby gift are good enough." If you had a different medical complication of childbirth, such as postpartum anemia or an infection, you would not impose this standard on yourself.

Is it *restlessness*? Do you try but fail to sleep during your baby's nap? Do you just lie there and worry? If so, try letting go by changing your expectations. Try for rest rather than sleep. Take a warm bubble bath during this time, or put your feet up and watch a soap opera.

Is it *unrealistic expectations*? Do you tell yourself: "I need to have my house as clean as it used to be"? If so, try letting go by giving yourself a temporary reprieve. Allow yourself to be a slob for two more months, or hire someone from the outside for a few months.

If you can't sleep during the afternoon, consider whether caffeine could be the culprit. Do you drink coffee, tea, or colas that contain caffeine? It doesn't take much—as little as one cup—to aggravate insomnia when you have PPD.

### POSTPARTUM ANXIETY INSOMNIA: "INITIAL INSOMNIA"

Initial insomnia only affects the beginning of the night's sleep—once you fall asleep, you generally stay asleep (until the baby wakes you, anyway). While initial insomnia may be seen in any postpartum disorder, it is especially difficult for some women with postpartum panic to fall asleep. In these cases, the sensation of drowsiness may trigger feelings of being out of control or even of having a panic attack, and the women essentially become afraid of falling asleep.

Oftentimes, initial insomnia is due to an inability to reach even a state of drowsiness. If you constantly feel anxious, you are operating in a chronic overcharged state, like an engine running at high speed all the time. It can be very hard to switch the engine off suddenly. You may be having a symptom called *rumination*, in which you cannot stop obsessing and worrying about things, whether large or small. This is common in PPD.

Initial insomnia can take on a life of its own, becoming an endless cycle in which the more trouble you have falling asleep, the more trouble you have falling asleep. This is called *conditioned insomnia*: eventually, when you can't fall asleep, your mind develops the expectation that you won't fall asleep, which in turn prevents you from falling asleep. It's a physiologic self-fulfilling prophecy. Much of what we will suggest is designed to interrupt this conditioning.

Look over this list of suggestions and pick the ones that suit you. Try them by themselves or in combination.

- Never lie tossing and turning in bed for longer than ten or fifteen minutes. If you haven't fallen asleep by then, get out of bed for at least another fifteen to thirty minutes before trying again. This interrupts the conditioned insomnia by deprogramming your mind from expecting you not to sleep in bed.

◉ Have something in mind to do if you are unable to fall asleep after ten or fifteen minutes. We suggest going into the living room and reading or watching TV for a period of time. This may actually be the best time to do the baby's laundry that we've been telling you to avoid!

◉ There's an old saying about conditioned insomnia: "Your bed should only be used for sleeping or making love." We would add nursing your baby, also, or cuddling up with your toddler to read stories. Otherwise, forget it; you won't be able to sleep. Again, if your mind thinks it's permitted to sew, read, watch TV, talk on the phone, and so forth, in bed, it will also think it's permitted to toss and turn.

◉ Establish a new bedtime ritual. For example:

- Treat yourself to a bedtime snack. Warm milk is tried and true (not cocoa—it has caffeine). Alternatives include herb teas or hot cider. Foods high in complex carbohydrates, such as whole-wheat toast or an oat bran muffin, promote drowsiness (similar to the early afternoon slump that follows lunch).

- Milk and toast is a perfect combination, since the tryptophan in milk may increase serotonin in the brain.

- Take a very hot bubble bath or a shower. The key here is to make it part of the routine. A snack, a bath, and then to bed.

- Once in bed, try a relaxation CD (as described in Chapter 4). You can listen to music, borrow an audio CD from the library, or buy one online. The use of headphones (as compared to listening to the radio) is a very effective way to shut down the process of rumination, because it prevents outside noise from distracting you. You may need to go through your

ritual two, or even three, times per night at first. Try
to stick it out until you recondition yourself.

- Exercise has been shown to help with initial insomnia.
  However, exercise can keep you up if done just before bedtime. Exercising at least several hours before bedtime may
  be very beneficial (even working out as early as first thing
  in the morning can improve your sleep fourteen or more
  hours later).
- A massage just before bedtime from your husband can be
  very relaxing.
- Consider temporary use of a sleeping pill (usually only if
  you are not nursing, and always under a doctor's supervision). While we don't suggest using a sleeping pill as a
  crutch for insomnia (because it eventually stops working,
  or it becomes absolutely impossible to sleep without it),
  temporary and time-limited use of a sleeping pill may be a
  crucial part of your recovery. To read more about medications for sleep, see Chapter 6.

### POSTPARTUM LATE INSOMNIA: EARLY-MORNING WAKENING

In early-morning wakening, you typically fall right to sleep but spontaneously wake up two to four hours later. This is not the same thing
as having trouble falling back to sleep once awakened by the baby. If
you are having trouble falling asleep at 2:00 a.m. after a nighttime
feeding, you probably do not have late insomnia, and you should use
the same techniques for this pattern as for initial insomnia.

Early-morning wakening is usually a sign of a more severe episode
of PPD. The good news is that it often means that medication is likely
to be beneficial, and it is one of the key symptoms that a psychiatrist considers in recommending antidepressant medication for PPD.
Even if the thought of medication does not thrill you, it should be

a relief to know that your symptoms are likely to respond well to it! The bad news is that changing your sleep behaviors, as described in the previous section, is unlikely to help unless combined with taking medication.

### YOU CAN'T STOP SLEEPING

One rare sleep symptom that may also signal a need for medication is extreme hypersomnia, the opposite of insomnia. In PPD-related hypersomnia, you may sleep for twelve, fourteen, or even sixteen hours per day. This is not the same thing as staying in bed all day due to fatigue, exhaustion, or immobilization. Hypersomnia means actually sleeping much more than your usual amount. Like early-morning wakening, it is usually only seen in severe cases of PPD.

## Nurturing the Nurturer

Most women are discharged from the hospital within twenty-four to seventy-two hours after giving birth and usually don't see their doctor until the six-week checkup. There is hardly time for a woman to recuperate before she is thrust into the throes of motherhood, often without the support of nearby family members. Although there is much fuss about the baby's initial adjustment and the baby's physical needs, there seems to be an expectation that the mother will run on empty for a while, that postpartum physical depletion just comes with the territory. But all mothers, and especially mothers with PPD, must take special care to monitor their own health and well-being.

It is essential that you make your own needs a priority. Taking care of your physical self through good nutrition, sleep, rest, and exercise will better enable you to care for your baby.

# "IS THERE ANYTHING I CAN TAKE TO MAKE THIS GO AWAY?"

*Medication and Postpartum Depression*

PPD IS A HIGHLY TREATABLE ILLNESS that responds well to medication. Medication is not the only treatment for PPD and is generally most helpful when combined with therapy. However, the effectiveness of medication for PPD makes it an option we would like you to consider, even if your first reaction to the notion is very negative. Elsewhere in this book, we use the term PPD for any type of depression and anxiety following childbirth. Because postpartum stress syndrome (adjustment disorder) and baby blues generally should not be treated with medication, in this chapter we use PPD to mean moderate to severe cases of postpartum depression and anxiety.

## I Can't Imagine Taking Medication for PPD

For some people, the idea of psychiatric medication can be very scary, conjuring images of state hospitals with zombielike characters roaming aimlessly around a sterile ward. For others, it may evoke worries about addiction or lifelong dependence on a chemical substance. Some just don't like the idea of taking medicine on a regular basis. Others view it as a cop-out or weakness, feeling that popping a pill does not get to the root of the problem. Others feel shame or embarrassment that may be magnified by the fact that they are postpartum, because it feels like taking medication now proves that they have failed as mothers. Women who are breastfeeding may also think that they can't possibly take medication until their babies are weaned. If you are considering medication as part of your treatment, we know that this may seem very frightening, especially if you have never taken psychiatric drugs before. Later in this chapter, we will discuss specific medications and how some of them work. If you are already taking medication, or if you don't have any particular bias against taking medicine for PPD, you may wish to skip ahead in this chapter. For those who aren't sure, let's address some of your worries and fears.

First of all, not everyone with PPD needs to take medication. Even though one of us is a nonmedical therapist and one of us is a doctor, we both have treated women with PPD with and without medication. In other words, sometimes Karen refers her therapy clients to a psychiatrist for medication, and sometimes Valerie prescribes psychotherapy alone. We base these practices on a complex combination of factors that include the severity of symptoms, the individual's preferences, the response to other treatments or to changes in support, and the risk of side effects. Sometimes, therapy alone works quickly and completely, and medication is never considered. At other times, all the support and education in the world does nothing for PPD until medication is added. Increasingly, as antidepressants and other medications have become more socially accepted, we sometimes see women on the other end of the spectrum: only interested in medication, and not open to talk therapy.

Often, nonmedical treatment provides partial relief—a woman may feel somewhat better for some of the time, or improve substantially but not totally. Certain symptoms, such as loss of concentration, severe insomnia, confusion, extreme indecisiveness, suicidal thoughts, and severe feelings of guilt make it nearly impossible to work in therapy. Medication can stabilize these symptoms enough to allow you to invest the psychological energy that therapy requires.

We strongly believe that in severe cases of PPD, medication contributes to a quicker, fuller, longer-lasting recovery. But this is *your* decision, and one that you must make together with the professional who is treating you. We want you to make an informed choice, which is why we feel it is important for you to prepare yourself with as much information about it as possible.

## How Do Doctors Know When to Prescribe Medicine for PPD?

When we raise the possibility of medication, women seeking help for PPD are often surprised and upset. Their reaction is frequently based on a misinterpretation: "If my therapist thinks I need medication, I must be really sick!" This is simply not true.

Psychiatrists and nonmedical psychotherapists look for a specific pattern of symptoms that suggests that a given case of PPD will respond to medication. For certain symptom clusters (called *syndromes*), medication is effective about 60 to 80 percent of the time. Certain rare symptoms (such as the hallucinations or delusions seen in postpartum psychosis) almost never respond to psychotherapy alone. In contrast, postpartum stress syndrome by itself is generally not treated with medication, because 1) psychotherapy is often effective, and 2) medication has no scientifically proven benefit.

Doctors prescribe medicines for illnesses that respond to medication, whether the illness is really bad or not. For example, if bacteria such as strep cause a sore throat, the doctor will prescribe an antibiotic, because it generally will speed recovery and prevent complication. However, if a virus is the cause of the sore throat, the doctor doesn't prescribe medicine, because there is no effective medication. To you, the sore throat feels exactly the same, but the decision to medicate one and not the other is based on effectiveness. Psychiatric illnesses are similar: some extremely severe disorders respond poorly or not at all to medication, while other relatively more mild illnesses respond well to medication.

## How to Find an Expert in Prescribing for PPD

In general, we believe that you are your best health advocate. You may need to talk with or meet more than one doctor before you find someone you trust. These principles will be discussed further in the context of finding a therapist in Chapter 7.

Many women first turn to their obstetrician, family physician, or nurse-midwife for a prescription. Often times, these clinicians are quite skilled and knowledgeable about prescribing typical doses of medications for PPD. If a specialist is needed, your obstetrician, midwife, or family physician almost certainly can give you a referral to a psychiatrist, or a psychiatric nurse-practitioner. Some women have a preference to receive medication from the obstetrician they know and trust; other women want to see a specialist right away.

There are times when you should consult a psychiatrist. If you have emergency symptoms such as suicidal thoughts or hallucinations, you should see a psychiatrist. If you have a past diagnosis of bipolar disorder, or if you have a sibling or parent with bipolar disorder, you should see a specialist (because sometimes the medications for PPD can trigger a manic episode). If you have been told you must stop nursing in order to take medication, we would recommend you get a second opinion from a specialist, preferably a PPD specialist. If you have not responded at all to medication after a period of four weeks, or only feel a little better after six weeks of medication, it's time to see a psychiatrist.

We also recommend that you take an active consumer approach to selecting your health professional. Taking an active consumer approach means going beyond picking a name out of the phone book, or choosing the geographically closest doctor on your insurance list. If you have insurance which provides you flexibility, do your homework (or let a friend or partner help you with this task). There is a terrific national organization that often can provide you with a list of local mental-health professionals who specialize in PPD. Postpartum Support International (www.postpartum.net) has a list of volunteers who serve as state coordinators. The website has links to the state coordinators that you can use to send an email inquiring about a list of local specialists. If no psychiatrists are listed for your area, contact one of the social workers or psychologists on the list and ask her/him to recommend a psychiatrist for PPD. If you are already in talk therapy, your therapist may be able to make a recommendation. Your obstetrician may also be able to suggest a psychiatrist. Support groups are an excellent source of referrals to a competent psychiatrist, and this is yet another reason to join a PPD support group if there is one in your area.

The following is a list of some of the PPD symptoms that may prompt your therapist or doctor to recommend medication. These include symptoms that suggest that medication is likely to help you, and symptoms that are unlikely to resolve with therapy alone.

*Symptoms Associated with Positive Response to Medication*
- Significant weight loss (beyond that expected after childbirth)
- Depression that is worse in the morning (*diurnal variation*)
- Agitation
- Inability to get out of bed or sleeping all day

- Extreme indecisiveness (e.g., it takes an hour to decide what to wear in the morning)
- Waking often in the middle of the night, even when the baby is asleep
- Suicidal thoughts
- Medication helped you in the past during a similar episode
- Clear-cut change in your personality
- Severe irritability, with frequent loss of control over temper or outbursts at loved ones when you previously had good control
- A blood relative of yours was helped by medication for depression
- Panic attacks
- Symptoms never go away—you never feel happy or take pleasure in life, all day, every day
- Horrifying thoughts or images
- Hallucinations or delusions

## I Can Think of 100 Reasons Not to Take Psychiatric Drugs

Some women resist taking medication even when they have very severe cases of PPD. The most common reason breastfeeding mothers are afraid to take medication is concern about whether it is safe for the baby. We address this important topic later in this chapter. For others, fear of medication is caused by an earlier experience that left them seeing a trial of psychiatric medication as a risk rather than as an opportunity, or perhaps due to stereotypes about mental illness.

Some women have had prior bad experiences with psychiatric medication, or know someone who has. Their concern is usually about the side effects, including the possibility that they will be "too zonked" to take care of their children. Fortunately, these days, new psychiatric medications are generally well tolerated, even in new mothers who require a high level of alertness to function.

Others are so sensitive to criticism that they cannot face the risk that someone in their life will not support a decision to take medication. They are afraid of being labeled "crazy" or "psychotic" or accused of having a "nervous breakdown." These apprehensions are quite common. This sensitivity to criticism by others may actually have contributed to your vulnerability to PPD, which means it will be necessary to do what feels right to *you* in order to recover. You have the right to feel good and do not need anyone's permission about how you get there.

Growing up in unpredictable or highly critical families leaves some women "control freaks." If remaining in control is a major concern for you, psychiatric medication may leave you feeling powerless or weak because you couldn't "handle" this on your own. This may include a fear that medication will lead to hospitalization. In fact, because PPD causes such havoc, effective medication will put you back in control.

Sometimes, concern about psychiatric medication reflects shame about having an emotional or psychological illness. Many Americans still consider depression to be a personal weakness rather than a disease—just remember how Tom Cruise responded when Brooke Shields disclosed that she had taken Paxil for PPD. If you or someone whose opinion you really care about considers PPD to be a personal weakness, taking medication may seem like another failure. We consider PPD to be a real disease, similar to other medical diseases. Ask yourself: Would I resist a treatment recommended to me for heart disease, epilepsy, vitamin deficiency, or an infection? Am I still blaming myself for having this PPD?

Embarrassment about taking psychiatric medication is extremely common. In our culture, it sometimes seems that we believe in medication for almost every condition except psychological ones, perhaps because we still haven't erased the stigma of mental illness. Some women find that a PPD support group can be very reassuring. It may help to see "ordinary" women who are recovering or have recovered from PPD with the help of medication. Remember, you can take medication even if you feel ashamed. It's private, and others don't have to know or approve. One woman reported that her embarrassment dissolved once the medication worked—only then was she truly convinced that this was a real illness, because it got better with biologic treatment. Sometimes talking to someone, in a support group for example, who has taken psychiatric medication, recovered, and gone off the medication helps ease fears of losing control or having a personality change from this kind of treatment.

## PSYCHIATRIC MEDICATION

*Psychiatric medication* is the term we use to describe medications that cause changes in brain chemistry that lead to changes in an individual's mood, thought processes, or behavior. The most common medications used in PPD are antidepressants and benzodiazepines (antianxiety drugs). Other psychiatric medications sometimes used include sleeping pills, mood stabilizers and antipsychotic drugs. We will tell you about each of these types of medications and will review common dosages and side effects.

Please be aware that this chapter reflects the practices of one psychiatrist. The guidelines suggested here are based on Valerie's training and experience and are included as a reference for you, not as a commandment. Valerie was reminded of this when, during a talk about the use of psychiatric medication in PPD, she stated emphatically: "I never prescribe amitriptyline for PPD, because it has so many side effects." As it happened, there were two women in the room whose PPD had responded completely to amitriptyline, without any of the intolerable side effects Valerie had often seen. Each individual responds uniquely. The following are general recommendations that may or may not apply to you, but that you should have available as background information when you discuss the option of medication with your doctor. This information is not a substitute for individual medical advice.

We cannot possibly list every side effect for every psychiatric drug, so we have described the most common ones. If you are uncertain about any possible side effect, please ask your doctor, or talk with your pharmacist. If your doctor "doesn't want to be bothered," please find a new doctor. Just as you have the right to ask for support from your husband, your family, and your friends, you have the right to discuss whatever concerns you have with your doctor. A doctor who isn't responsive to problematic side effects isn't worth your time.

## Brain Functioning

In order to understand how psychiatric medication works in PPD, it is helpful to know some basics about brain functioning. The brain is made up of nerve cells, called neurons, which communicate with each other through chemicals called neurotransmitters. Hormones help regulate the neurotransmitters. Imbalances in these neurotransmitters can cause faulty communication between neurons. This results in disturbance of brain functioning, which, if it occurs in certain parts of the brain, we may experience as changes in our mood, thoughts, perceptions, and behavior. Since our mood is also influenced by life experiences, the intensity of symptoms may depend in part on whether the environment is stressful or supportive.

What happens to brain functioning in PPD? No one knows for certain, although researchers are trying to find out. The most likely explanation is that during pregnancy, levels of hormones like estrogen, progesterone, and cortisol are much higher than in the nonpregnant state. When the baby is born, these hormone levels fall drastically. In some women, this sudden change may disturb the balance of the neurotransmitters that the hormones regulate. In other women, sleep deprivation may trigger the neurotransmitter imbalance.

What effect will this imbalance have? Again, we don't know for certain, but it seems to depend on which neurotransmitter is affected the most. Imbalances of serotonin and norepinephrine may lead to depression; imbalance of gamma-amino-butyric acid (GABA for short) may lead to anxiety and panic; and imbalance of dopamine may lead to psychosis. Medications work by restoring the normal balance of these neurotransmitter systems.

Many women wonder why we don't just prescribe hormone replacements if the problem is with their hormones. Unfortunately, while there have been anecdotes and occasional promising studies about hormones and PPD, we still do not have the science to tell us how to use hormones to correct this complex chemical cascade that leads to PPD. A major concern is that hormones, even natural or bioidentical hormones, come with a huge list of potentially serious side effects, including cancer, blood clots, migraines, and liver disease. Reproductive hormones may negatively affect breastfeeding and be risky if you became unexpectedly pregnant again. This means that there would need to be a clear-cut advantage of hormones in order to justify their higher risk, relative to most antidepressants.

Be aware that the US Food and Drug Administration (FDA) has advised women that there is no scientific basis to the claims that bioidentical hormones are safer or more effective. It isn't even proven that bioidentical hormones are, in fact, identical to natural hormones. There is a lot of hype and a lot of money being made marketing these products. Don't take medical advice from an infomercial.

But the most important reason that most physicians recommend antidepressants over hormones is that, for most women, psychiatric medications that correct the neurotransmitter imbalance work well. You deserve a treatment that works, even if your gut tells you that this is hormonally induced. You deserve the most effective treatment, even if it would feel less shameful to take hormones. The best way to treat postpartum depression biologically at this time is with psychiatric medications, not with reproductive hormones.

# Prior to Starting Psychiatric Medication

Many medical conditions can mimic PPD. A physical examination with a careful assessment of the possibility of postpartum thyroid disease or anemia is essential. Also, a careful medical history and examination are necessary to be sure that the medicines prescribed are not unsafe due to cardiovascular, kidney, liver, or other disease.

Equally important to selecting the right medication is the proper psychiatric diagnosis. Please let your psychiatrist know what symptoms you are having, even if you are embarrassed about them.

### ANTIDEPRESSANTS

Antidepressants fall into five categories:

1. Selective serotonin reuptake inhibitors (SSRIs)
2. Dual serotonin and norepinephrine reuptake inhibitors (SNRIs)
3. Atypical antidepressants (which have unique brain chemistry)
4. Heterocyclic antidepressants (many are also called tricyclics)
5. Monoamine oxidase (MAO) inhibitors

The following list gives both brand names and generic names for antidepressants. The great majority of women who are prescribed medication for PPD will be prescribed one of the drugs listed as SSRI, SNRI, or atypical antidepressants, as they are considered to have fewer and safer side effects. Some psychiatrists prefer to prescribe tricyclics for nursing mothers. MAO inhibitors are rarely used other than in a patch form, because you must scrupulously eliminate certain foods from your diet, which can be a stressful inconvenience and even life-threatening if not followed.

*If you have previously responded to a specific antidepressant, it is likely that you will respond to the same medication during this episode of PPD.*

## ANTIDEPRESSANTS

(Generic names are in parentheses)

Selective Serotonin Reuptake Inhibitors
*Celexa (citalopram)*
*Lexapro (escitalopram)*
*Luvox (fluvoxamine)*
*Paxil, Paxil CR (paroxetine)*
*Prozac, Prozac Weekly, Sarafem (fluoxetine)*
*Zoloft (sertraline)*

Selective Norepinephrine Serotonin Reuptake Inhibitors
*Cymbalta (duloxetine)*
*Effexor, Effexor XR (venlafaxine)*
*Pristiq (desvenlafaxine)*

Tricyclic/Heterocyclic Antidepressants
*Anafranil (clomipramine)*
*Elavil (amitriptyline)*
*Norpramin (desipramine)*
*Pamelor, Aventyl (nortriptyline)*
*Sinequan, Adapin (doxepin)*
*Tofranil (imipramine)*

Atypical Antidepressants
*Desyrel, Oleptro (trazodone)*
*Remeron (mirtazapine)*
*Serzone (nefazodone)*
*Wellbutrin, Aplenzin, Budeprion (bupropion)*

Monoamine Oxidase Inhibitors
*Emsam (seligiline patch)*
*Marplan (isocarboxazid)*
*Nardil (phenelzine)*
*Parnate (tranylcypromine)*

## Common Features of Antidepressants

Antidepressants all have certain features in common; they differ primarily in the types of side effects they usually have. All antidepressants improve clinical depression at about the same rate—in other words, there is not a *best* or *most effective* antidepressant in general. It can be confusing to hear that one medication worked well for this person but not for that one, or that your friend recommends the antidepressant she is taking, but you didn't do well with it. There are a host of variables to balance when considering the use of antidepressants. PPD expert and researcher, Dr. Katherine Wisner says that *the best antidepressant is the one that works for you.*

Antidepressants are most beneficial in severe depression and may not be any more effective than a placebo for mild forms. Any specific individual may respond to one better than to another, which means it is worth it to try more than one medication if the first or even second one doesn't work. They all have a delayed onset of action—it usually takes at least two weeks, but often three or more, to show some effect. In part, the delay is due to the need to gradually build up the amount of antidepressant in your system. More importantly, the delay is due to a slow chain reaction set off in the brain called *downregulation*, in which neurotransmitter receptors are reduced in density in response to the increased level of neurotransmitters caused by the antidepressant. This essentially resets the system, which then needs to be maintained at the new downregulated level for six to twelve months. (We cover this more fully in Chapter 14.)

Antidepressants have a typical pattern of effectiveness. By four to six weeks, you should see marked improvement; by three months, you should have a complete remission. If not, a change in dose or type of medication is probably indicated. This can seem like a very long time, especially if at the end of this time, a new medication is needed because the first one did not work. Fortunately, most PPD responds to the initial medication. Because of the long delay, tranquilizers such as

Xanax (alprazolam) or Klonopin (clonazepam), which don't require weeks to work, are often prescribed in conjunction with an antidepressant in order to provide immediate symptom relief of anxiety and insomnia.

Most women with a single bout of PPD successfully discontinue medication within six to twelve months postpartum. The most common reason for stopping an antidepressant shortly after starting it is oversedation due to an excessive initial dose. Talk to your doctor about starting with a lower dose, raising the dose more slowly, or switching to a less-sedating medication. The downside of increasing very slowly is that it will take longer to reach a therapeutic dose, which means it will take longer for the depression to lift. You and your doctor should be discussing this issue if you are taking one of these medications.

The possibility of intentional overdose with antidepressants is always a concern for women with suicidal thoughts or impulses. For this reason, in rare cases, antidepressants may be prescribed in small amounts or only in a hospital setting until the suicidal risk subsides. The FDA issued an alert that you will see enclosed with your prescription called a "black box warning." Although this is controversial (and you can find arguments on both sides when you browse the internet), the FDA determined that any and all antidepressants may increase the risk of suicidal thoughts or suicide attempts in individuals between the ages of eighteen and twenty-four when they are first started (up to two months). They have not warned about increased suicidal thinking in women over age twenty-four. Most psychiatrists feel that antidepressants reduce the risk of suicide by treating the most common cause of suicide, which is clinical depression. As always, *immediately seek help if you start antidepressants and have thoughts of harming yourself.*

Individuals with *bipolar mood disorder* (also called manic-depressive illness) generally should not take antidepressants without also taking a mood stabilizer, because the antidepressants can "switch" a depressive syndrome into a manic syndrome. If you have never personally experienced a manic syndrome but bipolar mood disorder runs in your family, you should be monitored carefully and immediately report to your doctor any of the following symptoms that may occur while taking any antidepressant: hypersexuality, impulsivity, decreased need for sleep, bursts of excessive activity, irrational spending or buying sprees, euphoria, irritability, uncharacteristic talkativeness or pressured speech, and unusual religious preoccupation or increased religious activity compared to your usual practices.

It is important to know that antidepressants can have dangerous interactions with other medications. Usually, the most worrisome medications are used for psychiatric purposes (especially MAO inhibitors), so your doctor should be aware of this concern. Be sure to tell your doctor and your pharmacist if you are taking any other prescription medication. It is a good idea to buy all of your medications from a single pharmacy, since most have computer programs that check for drug interactions.

Some antidepressants aren't available in generic versions (Lexapro is one), are more expensive, may not be covered by your insurance company's so-called "formulary," or may have a higher co-pay than generics. If generics are available, Valerie believes they are equivalent. If there isn't a generic, or if you don't have insurance and finances are a concern (we know these medications are expensive!), you can sometimes save money by splitting a higher dose pill in half. For example, if your Lexapro dose is 10 mg, you may be able to save money by using a pill cutter to break a 20 mg tablet in half. If your pharmacy features a low-cost generic program, such as Walmart's $4.00 prescriptions, you should be able to get a month's supply of fluoxetine, paroxetine, citalopram, trazodone, and nortriptyline for between $4.00 and $8.00 (depending on the dose). Sertraline, the most common antidepressant Valerie prescribes for PPD, is available for less than $10.00 per month if you split the 100 mg tablet. Some nongenerics, such as Pristiq and Oleptro, may be far more expensive without any real benefit compared to their cheaper equivalents, venlafaxine and trazodone.

## Will the Medicine Cause Side Effects?

The honest answer is, most likely, you will have some side effects. This may seem like a very scary prospect. Fortunately, the side effects of antidepressant medications are typically very well tolerated by healthy young adults. Also, most side effects get better or resolve completely with time. It isn't possible to list every side effect, so remember: if you think you are having a side effect from your medicine, don't hesitate to check with your doctor.

It is often tempting to abandon the medication if it causes any initial side effects, especially since the benefits of antidepressants don't appear right away. Fortunately, side effects from psychiatric medications often resolve within days or weeks as your system adjusts, and once the depression is gone, any residual side effects may seem like a small price to pay.

Many side effects of antidepressants are annoying but not health-threatening. Try the following suggestions to alleviate side effects:

*Side Effects and Suggested Remedies*

*Constipation*
- Increase fiber in diet (e.g., oat bran, whole grains, fresh fruit)
- Natural laxatives: prunes, figs, prune juice (try mixing prune juice in orange or cranberry juice to make it taste better )
- Bulk laxatives (psyllium)
- Increased fluid intake
- Exercise

*Dry mouth*
- Suck on sugarless hard candy or ice chips
- Refrain from sugar-containing gum and candy
- Suck on a thin slice of lemon

- Ask your pharmacist to recommend an over-the-counter oral moisturizing spray
- Carry a bottle of water in a purse, diaper bag, or briefcase and take frequent sips

*Weight gain*
- Exercise: Join a mother-baby aerobics class at a fitness center
- Try munching on low-calorie snacks including unbuttered popcorn, raw veggies, or puffed-grain cereals; and avoid sugar and processed flour
- If you are nursing, please do not go on a strict diet—talk to your doctor or dietician to determine a diet that is healthy for you and your baby
- Talk to your doctor about possibly taking a different medication that doesn't affect you in the same way
- Consult a nutritionist
- Remember that part of why you are gaining weight may be because the PPD caused you to lose that weight you gained during your pregnancy too fast to be healthy

*Loss of sex drive or ability to climax*
- Give it time—this side effect may wear off within weeks or months
- Ask your doctor about possibly switching to Wellbutrin, Remeron, or Serzone, which rarely cause sexual side effects, or a tricyclic which has a much lower rate of this side effect
- Ask your doctor about whether a lower dose might be effective
- Consider taking another medication to restore orgasm

Be aware that sexual side effects resolve when you eventually stop the medication—this isn't permanent.

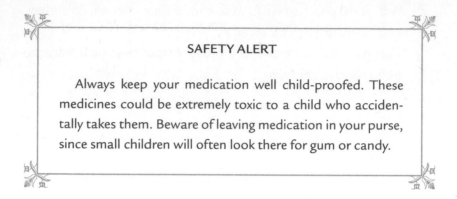

SAFETY ALERT

Always keep your medication well child-proofed. These medicines could be extremely toxic to a child who accidentally takes them. Beware of leaving medication in your purse, since small children will often look there for gum or candy.

## What Your Doctor Is Likely to Prescribe First

The antidepressants Wellbutrin (bupropion), the SSRIs (such as Lexapro and Prozac), and the SNRIs (such as Effexor) are most commonly prescribed these days. SSRIs are very broad spectrum, in that they help panic disorder, OCD, generalized anxiety, and "regular" PPD. Their main disadvantage is the possibility of sexual side effects, depending on the dosage. Since new mothers already often have low sex drive, this can be a very problematic side effect to live with. On the other hand, since new mothers often already have low sex drive, this may not bother them (as one woman said, "There isn't anything less than zero"). Since Wellbutrin doesn't have sexual side effects, it may be the best first choice for many mothers. There isn't a side-effect free medication, though, and Wellbutrin can make anxiety and insomnia worse. It doesn't work for OCD or primary anxiety problems. It also requires some time to adjust to the therapeutic dose.

Valerie is most likely to prescribe an SSRI or Wellbutrin for PPD, and feels that generics are equivalent. Doctors choose among these medications in part based on documented side effects and in part because of their own personal biases. Remeron and Serzone are also less likely to cause sexual dysfunction, but some doctors and patients prefer other medications, because both of these can be quite sedating. Remeron can cause significant weight gain, and Serzone has an FDA black box warning about the possibility of severe liver damage.

## SSRIs and SNRIs: Some Specific Issues

SSRIs and SNRIs have very similar properties. The most common nonsexual side effects of these antidepressants—if any—are nausea, diarrhea, headache, overstimulation (feeling wired or jittery), vivid dreams, and insomnia. Some patients find that they can tolerate a particular SSRI or SNRI better than another, even though these drugs are similar. Taking it in the morning may minimize the insomnia (most other antidepressants are taken at bedtime). In the case of overstimulation, dosage can be lowered to reduce side effects, or, for Prozac, the medication can be taken every other or every third day. Unfortunately, this may also make the dose too low to work. Overstimulation can also be eased by prescribing a benzodiazepine such as Klonopin or a sleeping medication along with the antidepressant.

Inability to achieve orgasm or loss of sex drive is usually the most troubling side effect of SSRIs and SNRIs. This is reversible when the medication is stopped, may go away spontaneously after several weeks or months, or can often be reversed with an additional medication or a dosage adjustment. Since PPD usually robs you of a sex drive, you could end up with an improved libido as a result of medication, but have a much harder time reaching orgasm.

When discontinuing any of the SSRIs or SNRIs, except perhaps Prozac (which stays in the body for weeks), your doctor should make a gradual downward adjustment in your dose. If you stop suddenly, you will likely experience an uncomfortable withdrawal reaction while your body readjusts to a new serotonin balance. The withdrawal can include dizziness, confusion, stomach problems, nightmares or sleep changes, or other unpleasant sensations such as electric shocklike feelings. It can also make you feel anxious, depressed, and even suicidal. This is called *SSRI discontinuation syndrome*, but it also happens with the SNRIs, especially Effexor. Unless you have an allergic reaction or have an emergency need to stop suddenly, you will have a much smoother ride if you gradually reduce your SSRI/SNRI when it's time to stop. You should try to avoid missing doses or running out of your prescription, since even missing a few days can trigger a discontinuation syndrome. This should not be confused with being "addicted" to your medication. Rather, it is the opposite effect of getting used to the medications—the process which allows you to overcome side effects is the same physiological process that causes SSRI/SNRI discontinuation syndrome if you stop it suddenly.

## Atypical Antidepressants: Some Specific Issues

Wellbutrin (bupropion) is an atypical antidepressant used to treat PPD. It has different side effects but is as effective as other antidepressants for depression. It is one of the antidepressants least likely to cause loss of sex drive or of ability to achieve orgasm. It usually has no effect on weight. The most common side effects are restlessness, anxiety, tremor, insomnia, headache, and agitation. If you have a lot of these symptoms already, your doctor may either recommend a different medication or prescribe a tranquilizer (benzodiazepine) until the Wellbutrin takes effect and the side effect wears off. If you have migraines, you probably won't be able to take Wellbutrin (but you should know that SSRIs and SNRIs often make migraines better). The most worrisome side effect of Wellbutrin is the low possibility of increasing predisposition to having a seizure. In order to reduce the possibility of seizures, this medication is not usually prescribed for someone with epilepsy, anorexia nervosa, bulimia, or alcoholism. It is also administered differently than other antidepressants, and it comes in a brand name formulation that is taken once per day (Wellbutrin XL) as well as in two forms that are generic, taken either twice or three times per day. If you are taking something two or three times per day, put a reminder in your cell phone and/or use a pill box to help you remember. Wellbutrin is approved as Zyban for smoking cessation—be sure not to take both Zyban and Wellbutrin at the same time.

Desyrel (trazodone, now available in extended release as the brand-name version Oleptro) is another atypical antidepressant. It is very inexpensive. Trazodone's main drawback is that it is very sedating. This can be beneficial for agitated forms of PPD or when insomnia is severe, but it is often difficult to take enough of it to be therapeutic for depression because the sedation prevents raising the dose. Many doctors prescribe trazodone at low doses (25 to 50 mg) at bedtime for insomnia, especially insomnia induced by SSRIs, SNRIs, or bupropion. To get to the minimum therapeutic dosage of 150 mg (or higher), you may need to adjust the medication slowly, which is not ideal in PPD.

Generally, you can stop Wellbutrin (bupropion) all at once. However, some women find that they feel very tired or want to sleep all day if they stop without gradually tapering. This is because your body has adjusted to the stimulating effect of Wellbutrin, and you may need to drop the dosage slowly to allow your brain chemistry to become readjusted to not having a stimulating medication present. Unless your dosage is very high, you can usually stop trazodone all at once.

## Tricyclic/Heterocyclic Antidepressants

The two tricyclic antidepressants Valerie prescribes most often are Norpramin (desipramine), and Pamelor or Aventyl (nortriptyline). A common starting dose for both Norpramin and Pamelor is 25 mg at bedtime, increasing by 10 to 25 mg every three days until either the side effects are bothersome or the total dose is at the usual therapeutic range. For Norpramin, this is usually 100 to 300 mg per day, often split into divided doses throughout the day; for Pamelor, this is usually 50 to 150 mg, typically all at bedtime. These two antidepressants cause less sedation than other heterocyclics, which is important for most women caring for a small infant twenty-four hours a day. There are, however, two drawbacks to using these two antidepressants: 1) Norpramin sometimes cause more initial jitteriness, especially if you have panic disorder, and may make insomnia worse in the beginning. 2) Pamelor, which usually helps sleep right away, can cause increased appetite and weight gain within weeks to months in about 40 percent of women. If you experience side effects, they may go away by starting at an even lower dose (10 mg) and increasing slowly while your body adjusts to the drug.

The most common side effects of heterocyclic antidepressants are dry mouth, mild drowsiness, headache, night sweats, increased appetite and weight gain, constipation, blurred vision, low blood pressure and/or dizziness when standing up, and tremor. Loss of the ability to achieve orgasm is occasionally caused by a heterocyclic antidepressant. Many of these side effects will go away over time or if the dose is lowered. If you experience a lot of side effects at a relatively low dose, or if you don't respond to the usual doses, your doctor may order a blood test to see whether the dose is in the therapeutic range. Antidepressants (of all types) are not addictive since they do not cause any "high" or euphoric feeling.

The most serious side effects are fortunately rare. These include allergic skin reactions, seizures (usually seen in those suffering from alcoholism or preexisting epilepsy), and serious cardiac problems (usually those with preexisting heart problems). One antidepressant called Asendin (amoxapine) has a unique potential side effect of abnormal movements after long-term use, so it is usually prescribed only in special cases.

## Monoamine Oxidase Inhibitors

Monoamine oxidase (MAO) inhibitors are rarely used to treat postpartum depression and postpartum panic disorder. Although they are

as effective as other antidepressants, they have strict dietary requirements, so they are not commonly prescribed unless one or more other
antidepressants have failed. These medications inhibit the enzyme
monoamine oxidase, which metabolizes neurotransmitters, including
norepinephrine and serotonin. Although the mechanism is different,
the result is the same as for heterocyclic antidepressants: more of these
mood-stabilizing neurotransmitters are available at the crucial parts of
the brain, and depression lifts.

The newer patch containing the MAO inhibitor selegiline is called
Emsam. At the lowest dose, this form usually does not require dietary adjustments, although the possibility of drug interactions is still
significant. In Valerie's opinion, only a psychiatrist experienced with
how to use this medication should prescribe it, not a general practitioner or obstetrician. It also is generally reserved as a second or
third line choice for individuals who have not responded to other
medications for depression. Its safety in nursing mothers has not been
established (more on this later).

## Antianxiety Medications

Medications that reduce anxiety (also called *minor tranquilizers*, *mild sed-
atives*, and *anxiolytics*) generally act to increase the activity of the only
neurotransmitter that inhibits brain activity, GABA. In other words,
these medications have somewhat the opposite effect of antidepressants, which increase brain activity. Benzodiazepines "quiet" many
different parts of the brain, and are therefore also used for epilepsy
and to induce sleep. Buspar (buspirone) is a unique antianxiety medication in that it affects serotonin rather than GABA, and it has no
addictive potential. All types of antidepressants except bupropion are
also used for postpartum panic disorder.

Benzodiazepines play a very significant role in the treatment of
PPD and postpartum panic disorder. One of their major advantages is

rapid onset of action, typically within minutes or hours (as compared to antidepressants, which take weeks). Women with PPD often benefit from taking benzodiazepines for a few weeks or months, until the antidepressant kicks in. Xanax (alprazolam) at a starting dose of 0.25 to 0.5 mg three or four times per day, and Klonopin (clonazepam) at a starting dose of 0.5 mg three times per day are often prescribed. Xanax has a rapid onset but also wears off within hours, whereas Klonopin has a slower but more sustained action.

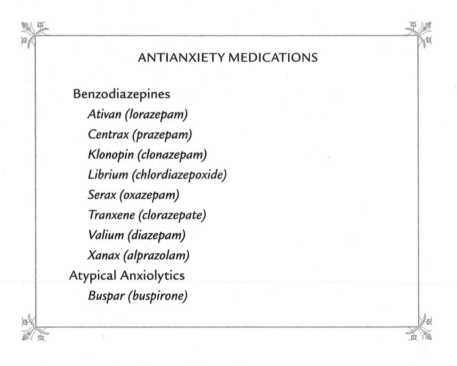

**ANTIANXIETY MEDICATIONS**

**Benzodiazepines**
   *Ativan (lorazepam)*
   *Centrax (prazepam)*
   *Klonopin (clonazepam)*
   *Librium (chlordiazepoxide)*
   *Serax (oxazepam)*
   *Tranxene (clorazepate)*
   *Valium (diazepam)*
   *Xanax (alprazolam)*
**Atypical Anxiolytics**
   *Buspar (buspirone)*

The main side effects of benzodiazepines are excessive sedation and light-headed feelings. This can usually be managed by reducing the dose, but it is very important to avoid driving or engaging in any potentially dangerous activity without being fully mentally alert. This may not be a problem if the medication is reserved for sleep, but be sure you are fully alert before driving. At high doses, clumsiness, slurred speech, and unsteadiness may occur. Benzodiazepines taken regularly or as-needed are effective for panic and agitation due to PPD. Buspar (buspirone) is not usually effective for panic disorder, and cannot be taken on an as-needed basis, since it doesn't work that way. Buspar is taken for generalized anxiety disorder, and like SSRIs, takes a few weeks to kick in.

The concern that women and their doctors have about benzodiaz-epines is that they will become addicted to their medication. Addic-tion or abuse of benzodiazepines can happen to anyone, but women with a history of abusing other drugs, such as alcohol, marijuana, or cocaine, or a genetic predisposition to alcoholism or drug addiction are especially vulnerable. You must let your doctor know if you have been treated for or are in recovery for an addiction before taking ben-zodiazepines. Buspirone is not addictive.

It is common to develop tolerance to benzodiazepines, which is what is meant when they are called "habit forming." The effect of a particular dose may diminish over time, requiring an increased dose for the same effect. Fortunately, in PPD, benzodiazepines are usually used only for a few weeks or months, and the antidepressant takes effect before tolerance to the benzodiazepines develops. When you no longer need a benzodiazepine, the dose should be gradually low-ered under a doctor's supervision, rather than suddenly discontinued. This is known as tapering, and it is done to avoid a rebound anxiety or rebound insomnia state, or even a physiologic withdrawal effect.

Some benzodiazepines can be used for anxiety or as sleeping pills, but some work best only for one or the other. The medications listed below are best used for insomnia, but are rarely used for anxiety. Ben-zodiazepines are useful sleeping medications when an antidepressant such as Prozac causes insomnia. Tolerance may occur when they are used every night, and sometimes a period of worsened sleep will fol-low discontinuation of prolonged use of sleeping medication. Most doctors try to avoid prescribing sleeping medications regularly or for longer than one or two months.

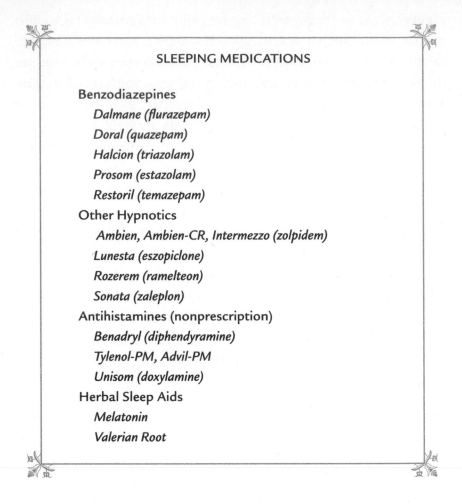

**SLEEPING MEDICATIONS**

Benzodiazepines
*Dalmane (flurazepam)*
*Doral (quazepam)*
*Halcion (triazolam)*
*Prosom (estazolam)*
*Restoril (temazepam)*
Other Hypnotics
*Ambien, Ambien-CR, Intermezzo (zolpidem)*
*Lunesta (eszopiclone)*
*Rozerem (ramelteon)*
*Sonata (zaleplon)*
Antihistamines (nonprescription)
*Benadryl (diphendyramine)*
*Tylenol-PM, Advil-PM*
*Unisom (doxylamine)*
Herbal Sleep Aids
*Melatonin*
*Valerian Root*

Increasingly, doctors are prescribing low doses of the very sedating antidepressants (most commonly, trazodone, doxepin, and amitriptyline) for sleep, along with another antidepressant such as fluoxetine or desipramine. The advantages are: no danger of addiction in predisposed women, less risk of developing tolerance, and possible potentiation or boosting of the primary antidepressant. Zolpidem is a nonbenzodiazepine sleeping pill that has an advantage over traditional sleeping pills in that it rarely causes sedation the next morning. It does not affect anxiety, but it also has less addictive potential.

The over-the-counter (nonprescription) antihistamines listed above are very mild, and may not work for the severe insomnia seen in PPD. However, they are often very useful for occasional (once or twice per week) use in postpartum stress with mild difficulty falling asleep. The usual dose is 25 to 50 mg at bedtime. The most common side effects are dry mouth, constipation, and occasionally blurred vision. Some women prefer to try natural remedies such as melatonin (0.5 to 1.0 mg) or valerian root (300 to 900 mg) for sleep. These may be very effective, or they may not be strong enough, depending on the severity and cause of the insomnia. Also, even though they are natural, they can cause side effects (such as sedation the next morning) and should be taken only after consultation with your physician. Valerian root has a very foul "stinky cheese" odor, so the first time you open the bottle, you may mistakenly think it is spoiled.

Barbiturates were commonly used in the past to treat insomnia. In Valerie's opinion, barbiturates such as secobarbital (Seconal), and the medications Placidyl, Doriden, Equanil, and Miltown have no usefulness in PPD, and so we won't discuss them further here.

## Anti-OCD Medications

In the first chapter, we described postpartum OCD, a specific type of postpartum anxiety disorder. Medications from the serotonin-enhancing antidepressants also can be very therapeutic for OCD. (Many of these medications also treat depression, PMS, and panic and anxiety disorders.) Only Anafranil, Luvox, Paxil, Prozac, and Zoloft are approved by the FDA specifically for the treatment of OCD, however, Celexa, Effexor, and Lexapro may be as effective as Anafranil for postpartum OCD.

Rather than list all the side effects again, we refer you to the discussion of side effects of SSRIs in the section on antidepressants. Anafranil is a tricyclic antidepressant (chemically related to imipramine), and has side effects similar to other tricyclics, as listed in that section.

However, it can also cause the same side effects as other serotonin re-uptake inhibitors—nausea, diarrhea, and sexual dysfunction, for example. For this reason, most psychiatrists try one or two SSRIs before trying Anafranil, which has more side effects.

Standard tricyclic antidepressants such as Norpramin or Pamelor are much less effective than the serotonin uptake inhibitors for OCD, but under some circumstances they will play a role in the treatment of postpartum OCD. Bupropion is not effective for OCD.

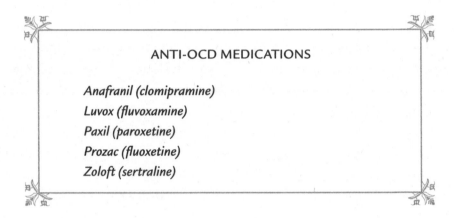

**ANTI-OCD MEDICATIONS**

*Anafranil (clomipramine)*
*Luvox (fluvoxamine)*
*Paxil (paroxetine)*
*Prozac (fluoxetine)*
*Zoloft (sertraline)*

## Mood Stabilizers/Antimanic Medications

Many women with postpartum psychosis will be treated with a mood stabilizer. Women with a previous history of bipolar mood disorder (or manic-depressive illness) or those with a very strong family history suggesting a predisposition for bipolar disorder are commonly given a mood stabilizer along with antidepressant medication, even if they only have PPD, in order to prevent converting depression to mania.

By far, the most commonly used mood stabilizer is lithium, a naturally occurring salt. Carbemazepine and valproic acid are anticonvulsant medications that may be used if lithium doesn't work or causes side effects, or may be preferable to lithium. The mood stabilizers have a delay of one or more weeks until they take effect. They are most effective for preventing mood swings and for treating mania, but are less effective in treating depression if used alone. All of the mood stabilizers require careful laboratory monitoring for blood levels and for possible side effects in the blood, liver, or thyroid (depending on which mood stabilizer is prescribed). Lithium may also used to boost an antidepressant when it has been partially but not fully effective, even if the individual has *unipolar*, which is the common form of PPD.

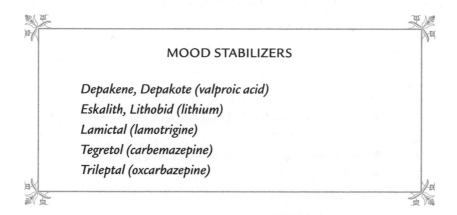

**MOOD STABILIZERS**

*Depakene, Depakote (valproic acid)*
*Eskalith, Lithobid (lithium)*
*Lamictal (lamotrigine)*
*Tegretol (carbemazepine)*
*Trileptal (oxcarbazepine)*

## Antipsychotic Medication (Neuroleptics or Atypical Antipsychotics)

If your doctor recommends taking *antipsychotic* medication, your first response is likely some combination of shock, disbelief, shame, or fear ("my doctor must think I'm really sick/crazy"). While the majority of readers of this book will not be prescribed antipsychotic medication for psychosis, for some women, antipsychotics provide tremendous relief of very distressing symptoms. For others, the new type of medication called *atypical antipsychotic* medications make the antidepressant work more effectively. You should discuss with your doctor why this particular class of medication is recommended. In current practices, low dose add-on therapy with an atypical antipsychotic is extremely common, and does not necessarily signify that there is something more serious than ordinary PPD going on. They also don't make you become psychotic, or indicate that you have bipolar depression. A key distinction is that the dosage used to augment antidepressant treatment is much lower than the dosage used for schizophrenia or postpartum psychosis.

Antipsychotic medications may be prescribed for postpartum psychosis, or for the rarer psychotic form of PPD. These medications alleviate the symptoms of hallucinations, bizarre thoughts, extreme excitation, paranoia, severe impulsivity, abnormal false ideas (delusions), and severely disorganized thoughts. These forms of postpartum emotional illnesses are very much less common than "ordinary" PPD and postpartum anxiety disorders, but represent the most severe end of the spectrum.

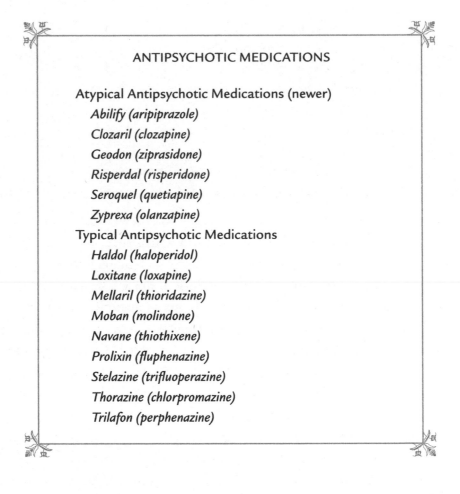

### ANTIPSYCHOTIC MEDICATIONS

**Atypical Antipsychotic Medications (newer)**
*Abilify (aripiprazole)*
*Clozaril (clozapine)*
*Geodon (ziprasidone)*
*Risperdal (risperidone)*
*Seroquel (quetiapine)*
*Zyprexa (olanzapine)*
**Typical Antipsychotic Medications**
*Haldol (haloperidol)*
*Loxitane (loxapine)*
*Mellaril (thioridazine)*
*Moban (molindone)*
*Navane (thiothixene)*
*Prolixin (fluphenazine)*
*Stelazine (trifluoperazine)*
*Thorazine (chlorpromazine)*
*Trilafon (perphenazine)*

Antipsychotic medications are thought to work by blocking dopamine. Dopamine is a neurotransmitter found in many parts of the brain, and it regulates reality-based thinking, aggression, sleep, and certain aspects of motor functioning. They work quickly and often provide symptom relief until an antidepressant or lithium takes effect. Although the side effects of high dose or older *typical* antipsychotics are generally more problematic than those of the antidepressants and antianxiety medications, they are often the only effective treatment for psychotic symptoms. In low dosages, they are often well tolerated, and can help with insomnia and anxiety as well as mood. The most common side effects of these older typical antipsychotic drugs include sedation, muscle stiffness, light-headedness or low blood pressure upon standing, dry mouth, difficulty urinating, and blurred vision. Some of these side effects can be prevented with other medications.

Atypical antipsychotic medications may cause fewer side effects than older antipsychotic medications, but if used for a long time or at high doses, they may cause weight gain and can even lead to diabetes mellitus or high cholesterol. The newer atypical antipsychotics are very expensive. Clozaril requires weekly blood tests because of a rare but potentially fatal side effect, and is not usually used for PPD. Older antipsychotics should be used only when necessary and in the lowest effective doses, because their long-term use may cause an irreversible movement disorder called *tardive dyskinesia*. If you are taking typical antipsychotic medication, you and your doctor should discuss this potential side effect and how to detect it. If you are taking the newer medications, even at low doses, you should have baseline and follow up testing for weight, fasting blood sugar, and fasting lipids (cholesterol and triglyceride). Valerie often prescribes low dose Abilify to augment antidepressants because it has very low potential for weight gain. However, Abilify can cause insomnia, and can also cause a feeling of muscle restlessness called *akithesia*. Many psychiatrists prescribe low dose Seroquel for augmentation, because it helps with sleep, but this is one where weight and blood sugar need to be monitored.

## Electroconvulsive Therapy

Electroconvulsive therapy (ECT), or electroshock therapy (EST), re-fers to the induction of a series of brain seizures under anesthesia. We won't go into the very complicated explanation of how ECT can relieve depression here, but since some readers of this book will have undergone ECT or will have it recommended to them, we feel it may be helpful to mention it briefly.

To say that the idea of ECT is terrifying to most people is an under-statement; images of *One Flew Over the Cuckoo's Nest* immediately come to mind. Despite its bad reputation, ECT has a valid role in treating post-partum psychosis and some rare cases of treatment refractory PPD. Treatment refractory postpartum depression refers to PPD that does not improve fully with adequate trials of two or more antidepressants at the proper dose. ECT is usually only suggested when someone has not responded to other treatments, because it requires general an-esthesia and hospitalization. However, it is the most effective treat-ment for severe depression. Since mood stabilizers and antipsychotic medications cannot be taken by a breastfeeding mother, ECT may be considered in cases where these medications are recommended to a woman with a strong wish to continue nursing. If it is recommended for you or someone you care about, we recommend you maintain a questioning but open mind. Unlike in the movies, complete muscle relaxation and general anesthesia are now used. At many hospitals, a second opinion recommending ECT is required and may be very helpful if you are considering ECT.

## Talking with a Psychiatrist About Medication

Sometimes, talking to a doctor can be intimidating—with so much at stake, it is easy to adopt a passive role and assume that the person in authority will tell you whatever you need to know. Even though both of us are healthcare providers, we know how often we ourselves have left the doctor's office forgetting to ask about something that concerned us. This often happens when your schedule is hectic or when the doctor seems busy. Being depressed or anxious doesn't make it any easier to be assertive.

Think about what your own mental obstacles to asking questions of a psychiatrist might be. Do you fear authority? Do you feel that your problems aren't important enough to take up her time? Do you believe that it is the doctor's job to decide what is important for you to know about? Are you afraid of what the answers might be? Are you used to doctors who are annoyed by questions? Are you uncertain of the ground rules or how it all works because you have never consulted a psychiatrist before?

Sometimes women are afraid that their doctor will be offended by their questions, as if they might be questioning her credentials or medical judgment. We feel strongly that you shouldn't worry about this. A good psychiatrist will want her patient to feel comfortable and be knowledgeable about her treatment. A doctor who is too busy, too grouchy, or too condescending ("Let me do the worrying, honey") to answer your questions with respect and consideration is not the right doctor for you. For all of these reasons, we encourage you to write down any questions or concerns that you have—about taking medication, side effects, or anything related to your treatment—and bring the list to your next appointment. You deserve to know about your illness and your treatment—ASK! You may want to bring someone to the appointment to take notes or ask the questions you forget. This is your right.

## Psychiatric Medication and Alcohol

A common concern about psychiatric medications is whether one can safely drink alcohol while taking them. We advise against all but an occasional beer, wine, or mixed drink, for a few reasons. The first is that alcohol itself is a depressant—it may make you feel worse and/or make your sleep worse. This sometimes seems to go against personal experience—we all know that one of the effects of drinking too much alcohol is falling asleep. Alcohol does induce sleepiness, but, as we discussed in Chapter 5, it also induces *middle insomnia*, causing you to wake up two to three hours after falling asleep. It isn't worth it. The second reason to avoid alcohol with medication is that alcohol and psychiatric medications magnify each other's sedating effect. In simple terms, taking one drink while also on an antidepressant or antianxiety medication is like taking two or three drinks without medication. Taking one Xanax (alprazolam) with a glass of wine is like taking two Xanax plus two glasses of wine. This isn't safe for you or your baby.

## Psychiatric Medication and Pregnancy

Pregnancy should be avoided while taking psychiatric medication for postpartum depression. For one thing, it is hard to recover from PPD if you get pregnant again too quickly. Also, while SSRIs are often used to treat depression during pregnancy, this is a decision best made carefully and cautiously. All of the medications discussed here have been classified by the FDA as potentially posing risk to a developing fetus, or lacking scientific evidence of their absolute safety to the fetus, so they should be used only when the benefits outweigh the risks. Since the first trimester is the period of greatest fetal development, early pregnancy exposure (for example, the first few weeks after a missed period) is of concern. For this reason, we strongly encourage you to use dependable birth control consistently while taking these medications. Relying on breastfeeding for contraception will not provide you the protection you need. The risks of fetal damage are small enough (the vast majority of infants exposed to psychiatric medication are completely normal, but it depends which medication you are taking) that you should not panic if you do have an unanticipated pregnancy—but do contact your doctor right away if you may be pregnant. (A positive home pregnancy test makes it extremely likely that you are pregnant. A negative home pregnancy test doesn't prove that you are not pregnant.) Medications known to cause birth defects include lithium, Depakote, and Tegretol.

Depending on where you are in your illness, you may be totally celibate because PPD has completely eliminated your sex drive. During this highly symptomatic phase, it may not seem that you will ever feel like making love again, and therefore you may not make arrangements to avoid pregnancy right now. However, as the medication takes effect, your sex drive may return all of a sudden (it often does), and you may be caught unaware.

Any available contraceptive method can be used safely with psychiatric medications. Sometimes, dose adjustments will be necessary if a woman chooses to take oral contraceptives (a birth control pill), especially with some of the mood stabilizers. While you are taking mood stabilizers, a birth control pill's contraceptive level may drop, making it less effective, in which case the dose of your birth control pills may need to be adjusted or you may need to switch to a different contraceptive method. Occasionally, the combined use of oral contraceptives with benzodiazepines such as Klonopin or Xanax may result in decreased metabolism of the benzodiazepines, in which case you may need a lower dose of the benzodiazepine. Some women with PPD experience a relapse of depressive symptoms when they take oral contraceptives, while others feel the same or even better while on them. This is just another sign of the complexity of the effect of female hormones on mood-related neurotransmitters. We advise PPD patients to watch carefully during the first few weeks of oral-contraceptive use for mood changes, and to try a lower-dose contraceptive or an alternative method of birth control if they notice more depression or don't respond to an antidepressant. Be sure your obstetrician or midwife is aware that you are taking other medications if they have prescribed birth control pills.

## Breastfeeding and Medication

The issue of whether it is acceptable to breastfeed while taking psychiatric medication is complex and somewhat controversial. Certain medications are definitely not safe for a breastfeeding infant. For example, lithium is unsafe because the baby can't always clear it from his system, and high levels may accumulate. However, most antidepressants appear relatively safe in lactating mothers, especially in light of the great benefits of breast milk for babies.

While the question usually posed is, "is it safe for the baby?" the real question is, compared to what? We know that it is not best for the baby or the mother to be clinically depressed or anxious. We know that many women would not consider weaning in order to take antidepressant medication. We know that formula may not be best for the baby, and may feel like a failure to many moms. Pediatricians are generally more knowledgeable about medications and breastfeeding, so if your psychiatrist advises you to stop nursing in order to take medication, we suggest that you check with your baby's doctor or your nurse-practitioner first—if they disagree, ask them to discuss the issue between them.

Most antidepressants and benzodiazepines are classified by the American Academy of Pediatrics as *effect unknown but maybe of concern* in the breastfed baby. This is another way of saying that we don't know that these medications are safe, but we also don't know that they are unsafe. Most doctors agree that antipsychotic medications, mood stabilizers, and MAO inhibitors are best avoided in nursing mothers.

Many doctors who specialize in PPD believe that in some instances, certain antidepressants can be taken by a nursing mother, provided that the baby's doctor is involved in the decision and that the baby is carefully monitored for potential side effects. Valerie is comfortable prescribing tricyclics, and considers sertraline the preferred SSRI for nursing mothers. Bupropion is also a reasonable option. She also uses very low doses of antianxiety medications for short periods of time. Since Prozac has a longer half-life (the time it takes to eliminate one half of the drug from the body) than other antidepressants, it may not be the best choice for a baby's inefficient metabolism. The complicated decision to nurse while taking antidepressants must take into account the theoretical potential risks of even low-level infant exposure to antidepressants compared to the well-known benefits of breastfeeding.

We are both very supportive of breastfeeding. At the same time, remember that even though breast milk is considered to be the most nutritious food for an infant, having a mother who feels good is also extremely important to a baby. Sometimes the only way to make that happen is for the mother to stop nursing and take medication. The decision to stop nursing may be very easy for some mothers and very difficult for others; for all, it is personal. It is *very important* that you discuss your feelings about breastfeeding with your doctor, as opinions on the subject vary and agreement between you and your doctor about your treatment is critical to your recovery. Don't overlook others who might be helpful in talking about the possibility of weaning—your mother, your husband, a friend, or a fellow support-group member.

Discuss the option of pumping your milk for a period of time with your doctor. For example, if you are having anxiety attacks or insomnia due to PPD, a few days or even a week or two of antianxiety medication may be extremely helpful. If you or the doctor feels it best to avoid nursing while taking antianxiety medication, you could pump your breast milk (and discard it), in order to keep your milk supply up until you can nurse again. ECT is another option for women with severe PPD who are determined to continue breastfeeding.

Some doctors are very familiar with the use of psychiatric medications in breastfeeding; others are not. This chapter is not a substitute for an individualized assessment and decision made between a woman and her personal physician. There is considerable information about medication in breastfeeding at the Harvard Massachusetts General Hospital

Center for Women's Mental Health (www.womensmentalhealth.org), which might be helpful to your doctor if you are nursing. They also offer a paid consultation on use of psychiatric medication in breastfeeding by telephone, which can be reassuring and especially useful for women without a local PPD expert.

Whatever your decision about breastfeeding, keep in mind that breastfeeding is not a test of how competent a mother is, how feminine she is, or how much she loves her baby. It is just one way that some mothers choose to feed their babies. If you have been enjoying breastfeeding, and you have to give it up, this may be painful for you. But be assured that your baby will be fine.

# ·❊[ 7 ]❊·

# "WHERE DO I GO FOR HELP?"

## *Getting the Most Out of Professional Therapy*

*I*T IS NEVER EASY TO DECIDE whether you should see a therapist. When you have PPD, this decision is especially difficult because your decision-making skills may be compromised by the depression. You may be feeling pressure from friends and relatives to "snap out of it," and you are probably telling yourself over and over again just to "get it together" like you believe every other mother seems to be able to do.

When we think about intervening in PPD, we consider many factors: How bad are you feeling? How long have you been feeling this way? How different is this from how you usually feel? To what degree is your day-to-day living affected? All of these questions, combined with your level of motivation (i.e., your desire for change) can determine if and when professional therapy is indicated. Unfortunately, resistance to therapy is widespread and can prolong the decision-making process. To illustrate, let's return to Lynn, who was denying the impact PPD was having on her life:

145

A few weeks after her symptoms started, Lynn's best friend suggested that she see a therapist. Lynn was shocked—her, see a shrink? No way. Everyone knows that they just make you worse, or only want to hear about how your mother screwed up your toilet training. No thanks! But when she couldn't free herself from her sadness after a couple more weeks went by, she started to get scared. Then a funny thing happened—a friend of her cousin's (whom Lynn barely knew) and Lynn's best friend's sister each called her on the same day to talk to her about their experience in therapy. Lynn was shocked—these women had been in therapy? They seemed so together. As the word spread in her family that she wasn't feeling well after the birth of her baby, it seemed like people were coming out of the woodwork to tell her their stories. She had to face it—her stereotypes about what kind of people see therapists just didn't stand up to the facts.

With her best friend's support, Lynn decided to give it a try. She spoke with three therapists on the phone and scheduled an appointment to see the one who sounded best suited to her. At her first appointment, she found herself talking to this stranger about surprisingly intimate things. For the first time in weeks, she didn't feel like she was whining or complaining. The therapist really seemed to understand what Lynn meant when she talked about how hard it was for her to do things that used to be so easy, like doing the dishes or walking her two dogs. Even though things hadn't really changed, she felt less alone.

At one time or another during their illness, many women suffering from PPD will consider getting professional help. Some women will decide to "stick it out" and resist the option of therapy. Others, like Lynn, feel relieved by their decision to get professional support.

There are a number of reasons why women with PPD decide not to go into therapy. For example:

1. **Sign of Weakness:** "I should be able to get through this on my own. Everyone else has a baby with no trouble!"

2. **Financial Commitment:** "I can't afford it."
3. **Fear of Being Labeled:** "What if everyone thinks I'm crazy?"
4. **Mismanaged Priorities:** "I just don't have the time."
5. **Denial:** "There's nothing really wrong. This will go away by itself."
6. **Generalizing Past Experiences:** "The last time I went to counseling, it was terrible."
7. **Lack of Support from External Sources:** "What would my friends think? My husband will never understand!"

Let's examine each area of concern:

**1. Sign of Weakness.** It is very common to view the decision to enter therapy as a sign of emotional weakness. When you have PPD, this notion gets compounded by your family's, society's, and your own expectations that it is natural to be a contented, enthusiastic, "good" mother, and that you should be able to resolve this on your own. You may fear that if you admit that you need help, then you are truly out of control. Actually, the opposite is true. When you reach the point where you can say, "I am tired of feeling so bad. I am not going to continue to let this [PPD] take over my life. I want to *do* something to help myself feel better again," then you can begin to feel back in control. In many ways it's simply easier to submit to the inertia and not do anything about it when you are feeling so bad. It's much harder to move forward and take action to do something about it. It is your *strength*, not weakness that enables you to take that step. Taking action on behalf of your own well-being comes from a position of power. You will know that this is true when you move in that direction.

**2. Financial Commitment.** No one will argue with the fact that therapy can be very costly. Combined with the financial stress of the new baby, the extra cost of therapy may seem unmanageable. But if you were physically sick or you injured yourself, you would go to the doctor. If you had a toothache, you would go to the dentist. If your baby were sick, you wouldn't dream of asking how much it costs or if the payment was worth it. For some reason, when it comes to the mental health of mothers, we feel it is dispensable, somehow, or negotiable. Or, worse yet, it doesn't seem to matter as much as everything else does right now. But, right now, everything else depends on your mental health. Be very clear about that.

Although the cost of therapy may at first seem impossibly high, take the time to investigate your options. Your insurance may cover part of the cost. Your therapist may be willing to let you pay over time, rather than all at once. Many areas have mental-health clinics or university programs with sliding-scale fees, where the cost is adjusted to your income. Going to a therapist may seem to be a luxury that you can't afford if you are already struggling to make ends meet. But if you have been feeling the pain of PPD long enough and find it harder and harder to get through the day, it is no longer a luxury—it is essential.

**3. Fear of Being Labeled.** Fear of being labeled "crazy," "weak," or "sick" by other people is a common reason why women resist going to a professional for help. Some women say they are afraid that their family will think they are doing something wrong or that a therapist will surely think they are crazy. If labeling does occur, it is out of ignorance, lack of education, misinformation, or fear; unfortunately, a stigma against mental illness still exists. It can be so self-destructive to be afraid of what other people think that you do not take the steps necessary for your recovery. Avoiding treatment will not make any illness go away.

**4. Mismanaged Priorities.** This one is very simple. *You must make your own needs a priority at this time.* It's hard to imagine finding time for yourself right now, but being able to do that is an essential part of recovery.

This is not selfish—your baby needs a mother who is functioning at her optimal level. Taking care of your own needs is a critical part of taking care of your baby.

**5. Denial.** Although it may sound cliché, acknowledging that there is something wrong is indeed the first step toward recovery. We hope that reading this book will help you accept that you have a real illness, and that you will begin to recover. But only you can know whether your PPD is improving. Is it? Be as honest with yourself as you can.

**6. Generalizing Past Experiences.** If you have been in therapy before and did not have a good experience, it will probably be hard for you to seek out professional help or to believe that it could be helpful to you now. You need to consider that you had a bad experience with one therapist. Can you consider the possibility that therapy with a different therapist might help? Later in this chapter we will help you find the right therapist and learn how to judge how well the two of you can work together.

**7. Lack of Support from External Sources.** If members of your immediate support network (husband, family, and friends) disapprove of therapy for any reason, their opinion will likely influence your decision. At a time when even the littlest decision seems impossible, it would be especially helpful to have support from friends and family while you make this very difficult one. But remember, no one else really knows how you feel inside. Ultimately, this is your body, your mind, and your choice.

The remainder of this chapter will be based on the assumption that you are curious about the possibility of finding a professional therapist, by which we mean a psychiatrist, social worker, psychologist, psychiatric nurse, or counselor. We do not discount the valuable support available through other "nonprofessional" sources, such as a minister, rabbi, medical doctor, or self-help support group. But the commitment to ongoing sessions with a professional therapist carries with it some unique benefits, such as experiencing the relief that comes from sharing the burden of your pain with someone who is trained to be objective, supportive, and nonjudgmental. Other benefits that are derived from being in treatment are the boost in self-esteem resulting from: 1) having a plan and making a commitment to being well, 2) regaining control over parts of your life, and 3) the feeling that this anguish of PPD will end.

## What Types of Therapists Are There?

The descriptions below show that there is tremendous variability among therapists. There are marked differences in style, training, geographic trends, and individual personalities, in addition to the differences in academic credentials and treatment methodologies. We could not possibly be fair or accurate if we tried to objectify these distinguishing characteristics in order to help you make a judgment about who would be best suited to your needs. The following discussion will provide an overview of the basic requirements for therapists in order to get you started on your search.

### PSYCHIATRIST

A psychiatrist is a licensed physician (MD) who specializes in emotional illnesses. All psychiatrists have graduated medical school and have completed four or more years of additional professional training. A *board-certified* psychiatrist has passed national examinations in the specialty of psychiatry. Some psychiatrists exclusively practice psychotherapy (talk therapy), while others focus solely on medication; lately, it is most common for psychiatrists to address medication only. Psychiatrists and psychiatric nurse-practitioners are the only practitioners authorized to prescribe medications. If you aren't sure what technique a doctor prefers, ask. A psychiatrist who does not offer therapy can refer you to a therapist. Likewise, a well-trained, nonmedical therapist will work in conjunction with a consulting psychiatrist in order to make the option of medication available to her clients.

## PSYCHOLOGIST

A clinical psychologist (PhD, MA, or PsyD) specializes in psychotherapy. In most states, a "licensed" psychologist has a doctorate, has passed a certifying exam and completed a course of supervised clinical experience. A psychologist with the title "Doctor" has received a Doctor of Philosophy (PhD) or a Doctor of Psychology (PsyD) degree. The main schools of therapy are supportive, cognitive behavioral, interpersonal, and brief dynamic therapy based on psychoanalytic theory.

## SOCIAL WORKER

A clinical social worker has a master's degree in social work (MSW), with training and experience in psychotherapy. A licensed social worker (LSW) has passed a state licensing examination in social work but has not yet completed his or her supervised post-graduate clinical experience. A licensed clinical social worker (LCSW) has a graduate academic degree, has had supervised clinical work experience, and has passed a national or state certified licensing exam. There are social workers who have an ACSW or a CSW, but licensure varies by state, so it can get a bit confusing. What's more, it is common for social workers to choose only one set of letters after their name, even if others also apply. For instance, Jane Smith, MSW, may or may not be licensed. So it's best to ask or research your therapist's credentials if you are doubtful. These distinctions may or may not mean anything to you, especially if you have a good rapport with your therapist, but the specific licensing designation may indicate the level of supervised experience and whether or not your therapist is eligible for insurance reimbursement. You can often check online at your state's professional licensing page to find out.

## LICENSED PROFESSIONAL COUNSELOR

A licensed professional counselor (LPC) is the same as an LCSW but is for professionals who received their master's degree in counseling or another related field (i.e., marriage and family therapy) instead of in social work. Like an LCSW, an LPC must obtain supervised clinical experience and pass a state or national licensing exam.

## LICENSED MARRIAGE AND FAMILY THERAPIST

A licensed marriage and family therapist (LMFT) has a graduate academic degree, clinical work experience, and has passed state-certified licensing exams. Most are required to complete clinical training in individual or family therapy, and some are required to complete 3,000 hours of clinical work before getting licensed.

## PSYCHIATRIC NURSE

An advanced practice registered nurse has a master's or PhD degree in mental health and/or psychiatric nursing. In most states, psychiatric nurses are licensed to practice psychotherapy independently and can prescribe antidepressants for PPD.

## PSYCHOTHERAPIST/COUNSELOR

A professional who calls herself or himself a psychotherapist is actually referring to the type of treatment she or he offers, not his or her qualifications. A psychotherapist or counselor may have professional training and certification or licensure as any of the above. Unfortunately, some may not. Although most states now require that individuals who practice psychotherapy have licenses, we recommend that if you have any doubts, ask the therapist to tell you about his or her credentials and show you his or her state license to practice.

## The Cost of Therapy

In general, psychiatrists charge more for psychotherapy than psychologists, who typically charge more than social workers or counselors. However, there are no studies that suggest that appropriate psychotherapy provided by an experienced and qualified practitioner in any of these disciplines is superior to that provided by another.

Most therapists have a fixed rate per session, although some may be willing to negotiate this fee. Although some do, many therapists who specialize in the treatment of postpartum mood/anxiety disorders do not accept insurances. Be sure to ask about reimbursement policies. Those that do not accept insurances will be able to provide a statement that you may be able to submit for out-of-network reimbursement. Additionally, many therapists who do not accept insurances will offer a sliding scale in order to make services available to you.

### FINDING A PROFESSIONAL THERAPIST

Refer to our advice for finding a health professional in the section "How to Find an Expert in Prescribing for PPD," in Chapter 6.

1. The following resources provide names of therapists in your area who specialize in PPD or volunteers who can lead you to one:

Postpartum Support International (PSI) (www.postpartum .net) has a map of the United States that can lead you to the coordinator in your state who can help you find a PPD specialist in your area.

The Postpartum Stress Center, LLC (www.postpartumstress .com) has a list of therapists who have received post-graduate training by The Postpartum Stress Center (PPSC) and who specialize in the treatment of PPD.

*—continues—*

*—continued—*

2. The following reputable websites are good places to start your search for therapists in your local area. Some may list postpartum depression as a specific area of interest. Others may indicate women's issues or depression:

*Psychologytoday.com*
*Goodtherapy.org*
*Find-a-therapist.com*
*Therapistlocator.net*
*Networktherapy.com*
*Therapytribe.com*

3. Look into whether a local new-mothers' support group or parents' resource center has a list of mental-health professionals.

4. Ask your doctor (or your baby's doctor) to recommend a therapist. Also ask whether your doctor has gotten feedback from anyone she has previously referred to this therapist.

5. Ask a friend, a member of the clergy, or a woman's health center to recommend a therapist.

6. Ask a PPD support-group member to recommend a therapist in your area.

7. Your insurance website should have a list of therapists within your network.

8. A Google search might just land you right where you want, so search for "therapist" and "postpartum depression" and then your city and state.

## What Makes a "Good" Therapist?

Keep in mind that the letters after a therapist's name will not be a reliable way for you to distinguish between a qualified therapist and a good one. Determining whether a therapist is a good fit is not always easy, but it is extremely important. What is good for one person may not be good for another. Still, a match between the therapist and the patient is crucial. Pay attention to how you feel. Do you feel comfortable and safe in his or her presence? Does he or she ask questions that seem to be on target for you? Do you feel like you can speak honestly to this person without feeling criticized or judged? Do you feel the therapist has a good understanding of your symptoms and provides information that feels helpful to you? Trust your instincts.

Below are some questions you might ask the therapist on the phone before your first session, or to keep in mind during the first session or two.

## DO YOU HAVE A PARTICULAR INTEREST IN POSTPARTUM ILLNESS? IF YES, WHAT IS YOUR EXPERIENCE DEALING SPECIFICALLY WITH POSTPARTUM DEPRESSION OR ANXIETY?

Women with PPD report that they feel much more comfortable right away if the therapist has special training, experience, or passion for the treatment of postpartum mood and anxiety disorders. Though training in this area is not sufficient to make someone a competent therapist, we generally feel that a PPD specialist is preferred if one is available.

Even more important than expertise in PPD is an understanding of what it means to take care of a baby, to be a mother. This does not mean that your therapist must be a mother, but rather that he or she is sympathetic to your experiences. Thus, though special training and interest is ideal, a therapist who is sensitive to the needs of women and who makes you feel heard and cared for may just be perfect for you.

If therapists respond defensively or resist sharing information regarding their credentials or experience, they may just be following the old-fashioned guidelines that therapists should not disclose personal information. However, we do not believe this qualifies as personal data; we believe women have a right to know who is treating them and should feel entitled to this information.

## WHAT IS THE TREATMENT FOCUS?

When it comes to the question of short-term versus long-term treatment, we believe that returning to your previous level of functioning as quickly as possible is vital. Treatment for postpartum mood and anxiety disorders should be brief and solution-oriented, focused on specific, achievable goals. The initial, immediate goal should be symptom relief and a return to the previous level of functioning. It's difficult to determine a specific length of time for treatment, since that is dependent upon one's particular goals and achievement of these goals. It's different for everyone. But the general philosophy of short-term therapies is to provide symptom relief and solutions to the current problem as efficiently as possible. Generally, this can be achieved in two to three months.

Short-term therapies that are appropriate for PPD include supportive therapy, cognitive behavioral therapy, interpersonal therapy, brief dynamic therapy, and group therapy,

### Supportive Therapy

Supportive therapy is an intervention that focuses on immediate symptom relief and support measures in an effort to protect and sustain you through the early phases of the PPD crisis. Goals are accomplished through reassurance, comfort, practical suggestions, empathy, and helping you marshal your resources and coping skills. Although supportive psychotherapy has received less attention in the academic literature, it is probably the therapy that is used most often by clinicians who treat postpartum depression. Studies have found that supportive psychotherapy and pharmacotherapy (the use of medication as treatment) were equally effective and suggested that clients and therapists prefer supportive psychotherapy over medication when treating depression. Clearly, the features of supportive therapy such as empathy and a strong therapeutic alliance are crucial to the success of the other forms of therapy described in this section. If you've been in supportive therapy, you know it is a conversation-based therapy that uses direct approaches such as praise, advice, clarification, confrontation, and interpretation to help you gain understanding. If you're not sure if this is something that would be helpful to you, Karen's book, *Therapy and the Postpartum Woman*, gives the reader an inside look at therapy sessions with postpartum women and can help you get a sense of what is involved and how it might feel to you.

### Cognitive Behavioral Therapy

Postpartum women are often plagued by a host of strong emotions, ranging from sadness and anger to extreme anxiety and elation. Many new mothers are surprised to learn how much these emotions can by influenced by the thoughts they are having. Cognitive behavioral therapy (CBT) helps a person have more control over the way they think and feel. It is based on the concept that distorted thoughts which reinforce feelings of depression can be modified, which in turn modifies one's mood and emotions. You and your therapist would collaborate to establish treatment goals and work together toward meeting those goals, often with homework outside of the session. In this way, this problem-solving therapy can help you develop specific coping strategies to manage your negative thoughts and distress. This approach helps you learn how to replace automatic negative thoughts with positive self-talk. You may also learn how some activities can increase your anxiety, such as watching the news or searching online, in which case you may want to decrease those activities to see if your anxiety reduces in response to this change in behavior.

In addition to focusing on cognitive strategies, CBT also focuses on unrealistic expectations and maladaptive behaviors that cause disruption in your life. There are a number of strategies that a CBT therapist might use in order to reduce the interference that some behaviors might cause. An example would be exposing a new mother to small increments of time with her baby if her anxiety was causing her to avoid contact.

There is now research that concludes that CBT is as effective as medications and supportive psychotherapy for postpartum depression and general symptoms of postpartum anxiety. One word of caution: CBT is a structured, active therapy that typically requires practice outside of the therapy sessions. Some postpartum women find that the demands of child care make compliance difficult. Hopefully, your therapist will be sensitive to this impediment, and the CBT can be modified to best meet your needs.

### Interpersonal Therapy

Undeniably, the transition to motherhood can create significant social disruption. Interpersonal psychotherapy (IPT) is another structured, time-limited therapy that focuses on problems in significant relationships and on how these relationships impact your ability to function. In IPT, you would examine your interpersonal relationships and explore the feelings that arise. You might focus on topics such as marital issues, role transitions, social isolation, and the demands of a new baby. You would work collaboratively to strengthen communication skills and facilitate better interpersonal relationships and coping skills. In addition to working on relationships and communication, IPT explores grief as a significant part of postpartum recovery, helping women identify and perhaps grieve for the normal losses that accompany this transitional period in their lives.

A study at the University of Iowa that focused on the mother's relationship with her baby, her partner, and her transition to the workplace, reported that IPT is a scientifically valid approach for PPD.

### Brief Dynamic Therapy

Traditionally, the psychodynamic approach (also known as insight-oriented therapy) enables the client to examine unresolved conflicts, increase self-awareness, and examine issues that arise from past relationships. Using the model of psychoanalytic theory, the brief dynamic technique draws upon the significance of early-childhood relationships and experiences and explores how they are affecting you as an adult, particularly during this crisis. Unlike traditional psychoanalysis, this is not aimed toward long-term treatment and can be extremely effective as a short-term intervention (six to fourteen sessions).

### Group Therapy

Groups have been shown to be a very effective treatment choice for many postpartum women. Groups can be time-limited and focused on topics, or they can be open-ended and unstructured. Professional groups are facilitated by a trained therapist, while peer-led support groups are led by other postpartum women offering their shared experience. Both professional therapy groups and peer support groups can be very helpful in helping you recover from PPD. The benefits that have been reported include reduced feelings of isolation, validation of negative feelings such as inadequacy and guilt, the value of psycho-education, and the encouragement of others.

Both CBT and IPT have been adapted to a group therapy setting. In fact, most of the research on group psychotherapy for postpartum distress takes a look at one of these two modes of group therapy. The research shows that group CBT and IPT are associated with a reduction in depressive and anxious symptoms and are usually more effective in doing so than the care that women typically receive if they are recognized by their healthcare provider as needing treatment for postpartum distress.

These short-term modes of therapy are not mutually exclusive—your therapist may use aspects of each of these methods. All of these treatment methods do have some common ground: the first stage of any therapy for PPD should focus on support—you should feel better during the session. The initial phase of treatment is not the time to explore your past or childhood extensively. We urge you to find a therapist who focuses primarily on today's issues, the here and now. Remember, symptom relief should be the primary goal of any initial treatment.

Some unresolved childhood issues, long-standing marriage problems, and developmental issues may clearly overlap with the urgent issues of this crisis. We simply recommend that these issues from your past not be the *sole* focus of your treatment now. After recovering from PPD, many women use the experience to launch into in-depth psychotherapy, in which lifelong personality, relationship, or self-esteem issues are explored. We enthusiastically support this when the acute depression is over and the timing is right.

## WHY DO YOU RECOMMEND THIS TREATMENT?

This question is very important! Whatever the specific answer may be, the most important thing to look for is whether your therapist is open to discussing your treatment. After one or two sessions, he or she should be able to explain in general terms what the goals of your therapy are, how to accomplish those goals, and how to monitor your recovery. If your therapist acts like this question is personal criticism, gets defensive, attacks you for asking, or cannot explain his or her reasoning to you, consult another therapist. Also, a therapist with too strong an ideology ("I only do 'X' type of therapy") may be too rigid to accommodate your unique and very individualized needs.

## Determining the Effectiveness of Therapy

You should expect substantial improvement by six weeks in therapy and near resolution of symptoms by twelve weeks. Since recovery is more complicated for women with PPD due to sleep deprivation and other child care—related factors, we add on a month or so to this time frame. If you haven't met your goals or if you are actually getting worse instead of better, it is time to consider a change in treatment or a consultation for medication. Keep in mind that resolution of symptoms does not mean that you will be "done" with therapy. It refers to relief from the uncomfortable feelings that were interfering with your day-to-day living that perhaps brought you into treatment in the first place. Treatment failure is not necessarily the fault of the therapist. "Good" therapists often need to change treatment modalities or consider new options when therapy doesn't have the desired outcome.

## OTHER SUGGESTIONS

Some of the women in our practices have come to us after seeing other clinicians. Many of them discover that these unsuccessful encounters have helped them zero in on what was really important in their search for a therapist. They offer these suggestions:

- "Try to find someone who has experience in many aspects of treatment—one who believes in talk therapy and who understands the use of medication."
- "I used to see someone who was more impressed with what she had to say than what I had to say. It's important to feel listened to, really listened to."
- "Look for someone who will be straight with you. It will not help if they just say what they think you want to hear. I always like being told exactly how it is. Then I know what I have to deal with."
- "My friend was seeing someone who she was very happy with, and she recommended I see the same therapist. Getting the personal reference helped me feel more comfortable right from the start."
- "It's just a gut feeling you get. Like going on a blind date, you can tell a lot from how you feel right from the start. If it feels uncomfortable, I wouldn't put myself through it again."
- "I used to go to a therapist who just sat there and didn't say much. It was helpful for me to find a therapist who was more proactive and actually offered suggestions rather than just letting me vent. I felt more in control when I left the session with tools I could use in my day to day life."

## Why You May Feel Dissatisfied With Therapy

Some women who seek treatment for PPD are dissatisfied with their therapist but are uncertain whether their doubts are valid. They may blame themselves for whatever dissatisfaction they may be feeling. If you are in the midst of searching for a therapist and have already been disappointed, see if you identify with any of the following reasons:

### "My therapist never says anything."

Complaints that a therapist is too passive are common in PPD. We find that postpartum women prefer a more proactive approach; one that helps her feel cared for and secure. While a direct approach with verbal feedback is important, your therapist also should listen empathically and not rush to provide advice or empty reassurances.

### "My therapist only wants to talk about my childhood."

A traditional psychodynamic approach is often frustrating. You need to focus on the "here and now" and work on immediate short-term goals in order to resume functioning. We encourage you to consider looking at what psychological issues from your past may have made you vulnerable to PPD, but this will be much more successful once the PPD begins to resolve. If your therapist insists on focusing on past issues while your symptoms are acute, we suggest you show this part of the book to him or her. Therapists who do not specialize in the treatment of PPD may not be aware that placing too much emphasis on past issues can impede recovery. If your therapist does not respond supportively to this information, you will heal faster with a new therapist.

### "My therapist says this has nothing to do with having a baby."

Women are frequently disappointed and feel utterly misunderstood when they are told that what they are experiencing is no different from any other clinical depression. We feel you have the right to be validated that PPD is different from ordinary depression because of the physical demands and the need to care for the baby, and the constant flood of social pressure to be happy and perfect. You are right to expect your therapist to understand the enormous stress involved in giving birth and caring for a new baby, and to listen to what you have to say about the impact of your recent childbirth.

## "I DON'T WANT TO BE IN THERAPY FOREVER. USUALLY, I FEEL FINE."

One reason many women with PPD look for a new therapist is because they view their illness as a situational crisis, not a sign of long-term pathology, as suggested by some therapists. Women are reassured to know that this *did* happen because they had a baby and that the treatment can be short-term and effective.

## "I WANT A WOMAN THERAPIST WHO CAN UNDERSTAND WHAT I AM GOING THROUGH."

Many women with PPD look for a woman therapist with life experiences that may make the therapist more empathic, that is, marriage and children. There seems to be a bias that if a female therapist is married and has had a baby, she will be more in touch with the issues of PPD. This is not necessarily so. Other women prefer to talk to a man, perhaps to remove the sense of comparing oneself, or they may just be more comfortable with a male therapist. It's most important to trust your therapist and feel comfortable with him or her, whatever his or her background, gender, age, and so on.

Understanding why other women with PPD have been dissatisfied early in treatment will help you clarify your initial expectations of therapy. After identifying some of these trouble spots, you will feel more equipped to make an informed decision. We encourage you to be an active "consumer advocate"—choosing the right therapist is a very important decision.

## OTHER POINTS TO KEEP IN MIND

**Trust your instincts.** Make sure you feel heard, supported, and validated. If something doesn't feel right, honor this feeling. You can check it out by asking questions or by sounding it out with a friend. It's important for you to feel good about the therapist you will be working with. A positive relationship is vital to the success of your therapy. If you have some strong negative feelings that you think might get in the way of your therapy, they probably will. It may be particularly difficult to trust your instincts because of how depressed or unsure you are feeling right now, but we are big believers in listening to your gut. It is especially important to trust your instincts if the therapist does or says anything inappropriate, such as make sexually suggestive comments. If this occurs, leave immediately—and do not go back!

**It is not your job to worry about how the therapist is feeling.** For instance, don't worry about whether she will feel hurt if you decide to change therapists or want to obtain a second opinion. These professionals are trained to protect their own emotional responses or ego involvement. You do not need to be concerned about how your therapist is feeling.

**Do you feel safe?** After one session—or two, or three—ask yourself, "Do I feel safe?" (Or, "Am I feeling too vulnerable and too scared?") Listen deep within yourself. This is often a reliable indicator of whether the therapeutic relationship will be a workable one.

**Do a Google search on your therapist.** Sometimes there are huge red flags that are in the public view, such as licensure status, so be sure you are going to a therapist in good standing.

Cultural expectations can have an impact on whether or not therapy is something that appeals to you as a treatment option. Different cultures have varied practices and beliefs surrounding childbearing, and some may discourage women from seeking medical attention for problems. Do not be afraid to explain any culturally significant factors to your therapist. She is the expert on PPD, and you are the expert on what your cultural or family traditions mean to you. Together these combined strengths can hasten and augment your recovery. Again, the most important aspect in the therapeutic relationship is that you feel heard and that those things that are most important to you are acknowledged and incorporated into your work together.

### YOUR RIGHTS AND RESPONSIBILITIES IN THERAPY

You are not just going to be a patient or a client. You are also a consumer with certain rights and responsibilities:

- You have the right to ask your therapist for clarification, explanation, and justification regarding treatment choices, goals, and course of therapy.
- You have the right to expect that anything discussed during the session is strictly confidential.
- You have the right to ask your therapist about his/her credentials, education, specialization, and professional background.
- You have the right to refuse to answer any question or discuss anything that makes you feel uneasy in any way.
- You have the right to confront or challenge your therapist if you are dissatisfied for any reason.
- You have the right to change therapists or terminate treatment whenever you wish.
- You must terminate treatment immediately if you experience or perceive any gesture to be intimidating, threatening, or sexually provocative.

## When Is the Right Time to Start Therapy?

The unfortunate paradox of depression is that the worse you feel, the harder it is to mobilize the resources that will help you feel better. The longer you wait to initiate treatment, the longer you will feel bad. You may have to force yourself to take one small step at a time. Tell yourself you are just going to make a phone call. No appointment, no commitment. Make the call, talk to a therapist. See how it feels. Sometimes a brief, initial contact can feel reassuring enough to motivate you to follow up with an appointment. You must listen carefully to yourself right now and try to make the decision that is best for you. If you feel poorly for long enough, you will know when it is the right time to get help.

## Should I Continue Therapy After My PPD Begins to Improve?

Some women recover from PPD convinced that their illness was largely "chemical" or "genetic." These women feel good about their relationships with people, have solid self-esteem, and are at peace with their decision about motherhood versus career choices. Others come through the episode of PPD admitting that they never feel self-confident, are actually unhappy about significant parts of their marriage, or cannot assert their feelings and wishes to others. If this sounds like you, then certain life experiences may have left you vulnerable to PPD, and continued therapy may help you identify and deal with those circumstances. We estimate that two-thirds of the women we treat for PPD remain in therapy after the initial crisis has subsided, and they continue to explore some of the following issues:

- **Loss.** Losses relevant to PPD may include unresolved grief over lost loved ones, past pregnancy-related losses, a friend who moved away, a mother who died before she could meet your baby, or a marriage that didn't work out.

- **Codependency.** Codependency issues may include growing up with an alcoholic parent or in a dysfunctional family where parent-child roles were confused and you didn't get the nurturing every child needs. Two classic books that we continue to find beneficial for addressing the needs of adult children of alcoholics (ACOA) and codependency issues are: *A Workbook for Healing Adult Children of Alcoholics*, by Patty McConnell, and *Codependent No More*, by Melodie Beattie.

- **Abuse and incest survival.** The elements of physical, emotional, and/or sexual abuse that may directly impact PPD are having had your feelings and fears ignored and not having had control over your own body. We see very high rates of abuse in the women that we treat for PPD. If you grew up in a critical or punitive environment, it is hard to feel good about yourself in any situation, and clearly these feelings are exacerbated when you have PPD.

- **Other forms of victimization.** Issues related to rape or sexual harassment, for example, may affect how you feel about yourself as a mother. Seeing your helpless baby may stir up some unresolved issues about your own past experiences of helplessness and dependency.

- **Addiction.** It is unlikely that you will recover from PPD if you ignore an active drug or alcohol problem. If someone you love has criticized your use of drugs or alcohol, or if you have wondered about this yourself, consider consulting a substance-abuse counselor or attending a twelve-step program such as Alcoholics Anonymous (AA). Most cities have women-only twelve-step programs and/or professional treatment programs, so don't let the stigma prevent you from getting the help you need. Chemical dependency is a real illness that can be successfully treated.

- **Eating disorders.** Issues related to eating disorders are often exacerbated during pregnancy and the postpartum period due to the fact that these disorders are characterized by disturbed body image and an exaggerated fear of gaining weight. There is evidence linking eating disorders with depression, which makes the eating disorder an area of vulnerability during PPD.

- **Divorce or severe conflict in your parents' relationship.** If your parents couldn't resolve their differences or argue effectively, you need to learn to do so now in your own marriage. You may fear being abandoned, or you may become "clingy" or be unable to risk speaking up about problems in your marriage.

- **Habitually unsatisfying relationships.** This pattern may be characterized by loneliness, an inability to identify or assert your own needs, excessive preoccupation with making others happy, and repeating self-destructive relationships. Additional problems may be manifested in difficulties with intimacy, loneliness, being alone (people who can't be alone and are always in a relationship just for sake of a warm bed), and communication skills.

- **Chronic poor self-esteem.** Signs of this are always comparing yourself unfavorably to others, preoccupation with issues of body image and sexuality, lacking self-acceptance, or feeling powerless in important areas of your life.

- **Significant conflicts about motherhood.** This includes struggling with issues such as self-definition, returning to work, unmet fantasies about motherhood, and adapting to the lifestyle changes of motherhood.

## Can a Support Group Be Enough?

The therapy we have been describing until now refers to professional therapy that may, at times, involve your husband. There are a number of support groups that are available for postpartum women who are experiencing anxiety and/or depression after childbirth:

### NEW MOTHER GROUPS

Many of these groups are formed through parenting centers and target the new mother's need for socialization, sharing, and exposure to other women with similar experiences. Usually these groups include some organized playtime for baby. We find that some women with PPD do very well in these groups ("I'm not the only one overwhelmed!"), but other women with PPD feel worse ("I'm the only one this overwhelmed!"). Either feeling is valid and will depend on your individual situation and the makeup of the group. We find that women who do best in these groups are women with mild symptoms who are seeking companionship and baby-related activities.

### POSTPARTUM SELF-HELP GROUPS

These groups are usually led by a woman who has experienced some form of PPD and who can now offer her experience and the knowledge she has acquired as guidance to help other new mothers get through the illness. These groups can provide enormous support and hope for the woman who feels isolated by her depression and needs support and validation from other women. It can be a huge boost to your morale to see other mothers who have felt as badly as you feel right now come out of the black hole to full recovery.

The best resource for postpartum support groups can be found by contacting Postpartum Support International (PSI) at www.postpartum .net. Their website can direct you to a state coordinator or support group that meets in your area. Support groups typically meet between once a week and once a month. Most are offered free of charge, but if there is any fee for these groups, it is usually a minimal donation.

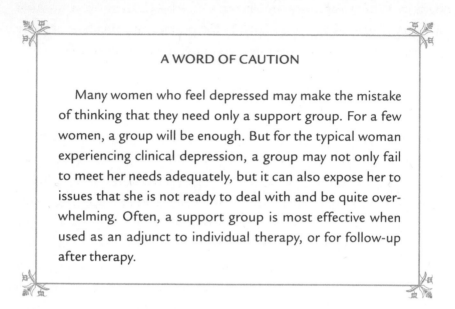

### A WORD OF CAUTION

Many women who feel depressed may make the mistake of thinking that they need only a support group. For a few women, a group will be enough. But for the typical woman experiencing clinical depression, a group may not only fail to meet her needs adequately, but it can also expose her to issues that she is not ready to deal with and be quite overwhelming. Often, a support group is most effective when used as an adjunct to individual therapy, or for follow-up after therapy.

## POSTPARTUM THERAPY GROUPS

Unlike self-help groups, these groups are run by a professional therapist, often in conjunction with individual treatment with the same therapist. The groups may be structured and issue-oriented, or they may be unstructured, with issues being raised by the participants. Therapy groups may meet weekly for a set number of sessions, or they may be ongoing. The fee is typically a fixed rate determined by the therapist. Many of the benefits are the same as for support groups—often, seeing a woman who is farther along in her recovery can be uplifting. But some women can feel worse hearing other people's problems or can feel too ashamed to share feelings in a group setting. Most women can determine if a group setting is something they are comfortable with, or if they prefer treatment that is individually focused.

## Alternative and Complementary Treatments

Although the newest APA guidelines (American Psychiatric Association, 2010) do not recommend any alternative and complementary treatments as first-line therapy for major depression, this is an area that is currently getting attention, and there is promising research on the benefits of these two treatments for PPD.

### OMEGA-3 FATTY ACIDS

Emerging research shows that low levels of omega-3 fatty acids are associated with low levels of serotonin, the brain chemical linked with anxiety and depression. Some good sources are tuna, salmon, herring, sardines, winter squash, beans, flaxseed, olive oil, and walnuts. Experts in the treatment of postpartum depression recommend the use of fish oil supplements as a safe treatment option for depression, both during pregnancy and the postpartum period. Although there are no FDA recommendations at the time of this writing, a dose of one to two grams daily has been shown to augment treatment with antidepressants. Always check with your physician for dosing instructions.

### LIGHT THERAPY

Like omega-3 fatty acid supplements, bright light therapy may be preferred by women who are interested in nonpharmacologic interventions. The investment is usually around $200 for a portable light box that can be used in your home. Though data is limited, bright light therapy has proven to be beneficial in the treatment of PPD. This is an extremely attractive treatment option due to the fact that it is easily accessible, well-tolerated, and safe while breastfeeding. We like it because it encourages you to carve out time in your morning to sit and take care of yourself. You can use the light box (typically for thirty to forty minutes sometime in the morning) at your computer or while having a cup of coffee reading the paper. Though it may not always be easy to find time for yourself in this way, perhaps it will be easier to justify it if it is "prescribed" time for exposure to bright light therapy while you relax!

## Making the Decision

The decision to enter therapy is not an easy one. If you are ambivalent about going to see a therapist, for whatever reason, consider finalizing your decision after going to one or two sessions. You can explore the option by visiting a therapist once or twice without making a lasting commitment. There is nothing irreversible about this decision. Remember that even though it is hard to take the first step, you can look forward to some initial relief from making the decision and following through with it.

# "No One Understands Me"

## *Getting the Support You Need*

$J$N Chapter 1, we described a series of steps that women usually progress through as they recover from PPD. By now, you have made some progress through steps one and two by using your internal resources and considering professional help. You should be feeling some positive changes in your emotions and your ability to cope. We expect that you have a deeper sense of acceptance that you have PPD and a better understanding of the symptoms of PPD. We hope that you have developed a few new ways of handling the stress in your life, have begun to set limits where possible, and have some new skills for overcoming negative thinking. Many of you have decided to get professional treatment for PPD, are in therapy, and may be taking medication.

While it may be easier for you to see the problems that remain, the bad days, the isolation, the fears, and the pains that are still with you, take a moment to reflect on how far you have come and to give yourself the credit you deserve for how much you have already accomplished. Taking time to note your progress will help you gear up for the work ahead. (*If you cannot see any progress whatsoever, please reconsider the alternative of seeking assistance from a mental-health professional.*)

The next three chapters will guide you through the third step, turning to others to help you make it through this crisis. Isolation and PPD are almost always found together in a virulent combination: each feeds off the other, and loneliness and despair spiral ever downward. It is imperative to reach out to others if you are to break this vicious cycle.

Family members, friends, clergy, neighbors, and work colleagues can be extremely supportive, and we will cover these relationships in this chapter. Your relationship with your husband is so important right now that we have devoted all of Chapter 9 to it. In our practices we find that husbands, bewildered by having a wife with PPD, don't instinctively know how to help you. Chapter 10 is written specifically for husbands to help them take an active part in your recovery.

## How Do I Know If I Need More Support?

Consider the following statements and check those that apply to you:

_____ 1.  I spend most of my time in the house.

_____ 2.  I have not made any new friends since the birth of my baby.

_____ 3.  I have lost touch with some old friends who meant a lot to me.

_____ 4.  Our families are supportive, but they live far away.

_____ 5.  I have not used any babysitter, except my family members.

_____ 6.  I know my family is trying to help, but sometimes they are just in the way!

_____ 7.  I do not feel as close to my best friend as I used to.

_____ 8.  Neither my family nor my husband's family is supportive.

_____ 9.  I seem to have lost interest in activities that are unrelated to raising my child.

_____ 10. I only have interest in activities that are unrelated to raising my child.

_____ 11. There is so much to do around the house, I barely go outside anymore.

Try to be as honest about these answers as you can. If you checked more than five, *chances are you are doing too much by yourself.*

Postpartum stress makes you vulnerable to PPD, so you need to try to reduce stress by asking for help and understanding. Perhaps you can relate to Marta.

Marta didn't feel like going to the mall with her friends and their babies.

She didn't feel like going to the playground to watch all the perfect mothers say all the perfect things to their screaming toddlers.

She didn't feel like going out to lunch with her mother-in-law, who had been asking for her company for weeks now.

She didn't feel like taking her four-month-old baby for a walk in the stroller, even though she hadn't been out of the house for days, and the weather was finally warm and inviting.

She didn't feel like answering the phone when it rang, because she couldn't think of any new ways to say she was fine but wasn't interested in doing whatever it was the caller was asking her to do.

She didn't feel like staying in her house alone. Again.

Marta is stuck in a downward cycle that will only make her PPD worse. Like many new mothers, Marta has disappeared into her home after having her baby and has limited outside contact during these first crucial months.

At first, Marta stayed at home most of the time because she was so exhausted—nursing every two hours left her no energy to get the diaper bag ready, bundle up the baby, get dressed herself, warm up the car, and try to zip somewhere before he started screaming in hunger again. But as the blues extended into PPD, she felt even less like going out, terrified of seeing anyone she knew. Marta was afraid that someone would immediately realize how awful she felt. But then, she was also afraid that if she told anyone, they wouldn't take her seriously. Worse, she thought they might find out her secret— that she hated everything about being a mother except for her son.

Marta feels trapped and invisible. She is afraid that she will be judged harshly because of her negative feelings about motherhood, but she is also afraid that someone might dismiss her feelings as being unimportant. Her fears jump back and forth between extremes: at one moment, she's sure that people will think she's completely out of control; the next, she's certain no one cares about her pain. The combination of fatigue, stress, and worries about being exposed or judged leave Marta feeling bleakness unlike anything she has ever experienced.

Marta has lost or cut herself off from what therapists refer to as "social support." Before giving birth, she was surrounded by people all day long in her job as a nurse on a busy surgical ward, and after work she enjoyed getting together with family members and friends. Like many women with PPD, Marta's isolation was natural at first— there was simply too much to do at home to make socializing a priority. But as her PPD progressed, the "think trap" that we described in Chapter 3 took over: What if people don't understand? What if my mother-in-law criticizes me? What if someone thinks I'm a bad mother? Not only can these negative thought patterns make you feel worse emotionally, they can cause you to withdraw from other people, adding self-imposed seclusion to the natural tendency to stay at home after childbirth.

Social support is a powerful factor affecting the severity of stress during the postpartum period. Earlier we told you that scientists don't really know what causes PPD. That's true, but one thing is well established about PPD: social support is a critical factor in the origin, course, and outcome of PPD. The lack of social support does not cause PPD all by itself, but it does contribute to a mother's vulnerability to PPD, and improved social support is a key part of PPD treatment and recovery.

Social support refers to the availability and accessibility of good relationships with others. Different relationships provide different kinds of support. For example, you might have an old college friend who you hardly ever talk to, but when you do, you know you can count on her to lift your spirits. Or you might have a neighbor whom you wouldn't choose for a friend, but you and she frequently count on each other to "just watch the kids for a minute while I run to the store."

Self-esteem and self-confidence plummet under stress. A support system can help nurture and maintain self-esteem at stressful times. In turn, high levels of self-esteem are linked with adaptive coping behaviors—feeling entitled to ask for help, for example.

## Ask for and Rely on the Assistance of Those Close to You

Relying on others means saying "yes" when someone asks if they can do something for you. It means allowing yourself to reach out for help and support when you need it.

### WHAT GETS IN THE WAY OF ASKING FOR SUPPORT?

A lot of women are used to doing everything for themselves, and that's exactly how they like it. But the truth is, right now you need to learn how to ask for help. If the notion of doing so makes you uncomfortable, because you believe only weak people who can't take care of themselves ask for help, read on.

Many women who used to enjoy the give-and-take of a supportive friendship find that the combination of being home with a baby and having PPD gets in the way. Like Marta, they fear being judged or are ashamed that they simply can't reciprocate any favors right now. If asking for help frightens you, stop and ask yourself how you feel when a friend or loved one asks you for help. Do you judge, reject, or belittle her? Think about it.

Women frequently find it much easier to give social support than to receive it. Even though it's an overused buzzword, women's difficulty asking for help is what the term "codependency" refers to: caring for everyone else's needs without regard for your own. Some women are so used to giving to others, they no longer even know how to get in touch with their own needs, let alone ask for help.

Codependency is a term for a very ancient way of relating: women have been the traditional caretakers in most cultures since the beginning of time. Society tells us it is feminine to support others. Think of traditional female roles: mother, nurse, teacher, secretary—they all involve being selfless, nurturing others, and putting one's own needs last. For some women, adopting the caretaking role is an automatic reaction, often a survival mechanism left over from growing up in a dysfunctional family. Being the caretaker is predictable—it puts you in control and protects you from feeling disappointed if someone lets you down.

We also know that being the caretaker often feels really good. Nurturing someone else is very gratifying and comfortable, and our point here is not to tell you to stop caring and doing for other people. But there is a time and place for everything, and right now you need to let yourself be taken care of for a change. You will be able to go back to giving to others again soon.

Having a baby challenges every new mother to develop new ways of relating to the world, one of which is learning how to develop and use social support. When this goes well, one discovers the pleasure of being able to take as well as give. Because having a baby is such a massive stress, it is often the very first time that the old habit of never asking for support is confronted or overpowered, and it may be very difficult to figure out where to start.

## WHO CAN HELP WITH WHAT?

Joseph Flaherty, MD, a social psychiatrist at the University of Illinois at Chicago, developed a specific research questionnaire that helped mental-health professionals define social support more precisely. Using Dr. Flaherty's Social Support Network Inventory as a reference, the exercises that follow are designed to help you break down your need for support into manageable components.

Part of successfully getting support involves asking the right person for what you need. Since the people in your life have strengths and weaknesses, it is best to target a specific need to a specific person. The idea of a support network is key: studies indicate that women with multiple sources of support adjust to the postpartum period more easily than women with a single source or none at all.

Listed below are particular kinds of social support that women experiencing PPD often need. Write down the name of one person who can meet that need. Try to avoid writing the same name down for each component. After you have filled in the first column, go back and write down one more person who could also meet that need.

| Need | Person Who Can Meet This Need | Another Person Who Can Meet This Need |
|---|---|---|
| Intimacy (sharing fears, secrets, vulnerabilities) | *Example:* husband | |
| Reassurance | *Example:* friend or therapist | |
| Practical help (child care, housework) | *Example:* sister, cleaning service | |
| Advice | *Example:* pediatrician | |

Now, at least once a week, choose one person from the second column of new people and actively seek out his or her support.

### Beginning with Practical Support

Start by asking your closest family and friends for practical, hands-on support. It may be as simple as saying "yes" when your sister-in-law asks if there is anything she can do. In our practices, we often suggest specific tasks that family members and friends can help with, and we encourage you to come up with your own. Some of the creative assistance we have seen our patients' families and friends contribute during a PPD crisis include weekly housecleaning (mother-in-law), on-call colicky-baby relief (mother), play dates for older children (neighbor), weekend or overnight baby care (parents), trips to the drugstore (sister), drop off and pick up at one of our offices (friend), an escort to the pediatrician (brother), and referral to a PPD specialist.

Here's one solution that Marta found:

Marta continued her attempts to act like everything was under control. When someone from church asked her to make something for a bake sale, she automatically said yes. Once she hung up the phone, she was overwhelmed. She couldn't face the ordeal of going to the supermarket, which meant she had to borrow an egg from someone in her building. After the baby fell asleep for a nap, she grabbed the baby monitor and ran across the hall to Jean's apartment. She asked for the egg, and then burst into tears. Jean hardly blinked. Her boys were at preschool, so she told Marta to go back to her apartment, and that she would be over in five minutes with a pot of coffee and some rolls.

Marta quickly pulled herself back together and tried to act like everything was okay, but Jean didn't buy it. Jean asked Marta what was wrong, and it all came pouring out: "I'm inundated with chores, at my wits' end, and haven't had time to take a shower much less go grocery shopping." Jean just rolled her eyes. "Why didn't you tell me you needed a hand? Just give me your list, and I'll pick up your things when I do my shopping!" Jean informed Marta that since her own children were born, she never actually made cookies for bake sales, and she ordered Marta to bring cookies from the bakery instead. Slowly, it dawned on Marta that Jean wasn't criticizing her for needing help. She was just surprised that Marta hadn't let her know sooner, as she didn't have a clue from Marta's carefully controlled appearance!

Marta never did let Jean know about the PPD, but a friendship began: Marta needed help, and Jean felt good about herself when she was able to give advice as an experienced mother.

We know it is hard to put any energy toward forming new relationships, when there is so much else going on right now. But the truth is, much of what has been discussed in this chapter would be applicable to any mother who is taking care of a new baby. This is not unique to mothers suffering PPD. Feeling isolated, lonely, and misunderstood are common complaints for parents in the postpartum period—even if they are having a second, third, or fourth baby. Remember, some postpartum adjustment problems are normal effects of the transition to a new family structure.

### Cultivating Emotional Support

It is often helpful to think about emotional support as having three major components: intimacy, reassurance, and advice. We don't see many new mothers lacking for advice about baby care: there are numerous baby books, magazines, television shows, and all too many people willing to give their opinions both in person and across the Internet, so we won't elaborate here. Women with PPD most often need reassurance about having PPD, and we cover this later in this chapter. Here, we will suggest some ways to cultivate intimacy, the emotional sharing of vulnerabilities that is a critical component of social support.

If you generally find it hard to trust people, you may have had significant life experiences that interfere with your ability to cultivate intimacy. In that case, the few words of advice we provide are not likely to reverse a lifelong pattern. Therapy would probably be helpful to you in this circumstance. However, if the isolation of having a baby and/or having PPD has interrupted or sidetracked your usual ability to find pleasure in emotional sharing, these suggestions are far more likely to get you back on course.

We find that the most common reason women with PPD avoid having a heart-to-heart talk with someone is that they gradually slip into a state of seclusion. As it did for Marta, home becomes their solitary confinement, uninhabited by adults for hours on end. No matter how gratifying your baby is in other ways, he cannot be a supportive listener!

Make a list of all the people who you feel you can talk to. Next to their names, list their relationship to you and what kinds of things you can talk about with them.

| Name | Relationship | What I Can Talk About With This Person | |
|------|-------------|----------------------------------------|---|
| *Example:* Jennifer | my neighbor | my husband | |
| | my sister | my relationship with our mother | |
| a. | _____ | _____ | _____ |
| b. | _____ | _____ | _____ |
| c. | _____ | _____ | _____ |
| d. | _____ | _____ | _____ |
| e. | _____ | _____ | _____ |

Now, as in the previous exercise, make a point of reaching out to one of the people on this list. Make a phone call and schedule time to be together, preferably in a place where you can comfortably chat. Going to the zoo together with your combined four kids won't work as well as getting together alone for coffee on a Saturday morning. Reestablish a connection with one person from this list at least once a week.

Isolation is a dangerous condition during this time of transition. Avoid surrendering to feelings of isolation—getting out of the house *every day* must be a top priority right now.

Many of our patients have had success with the following ways of overcoming isolation:

- Invite a friend over to watch TV, or take a walk together
- Meet a friend for lunch
- Join a mother's group
- Start attending a mother-baby exercise class
- See what is happening at your church or synagogue
- Go to the park or playground in your neighborhood and start up a conversation with another mother
- Bring the baby to your husband's office for lunch
- Join or start a babysitting cooperative exchange
- Attend a support group for women with PPD
- Put up a sign at the grocery store: "Mother of infant looking for same to start play group"

Think about the people in your life who you enjoy being with. Who is available to spend time with you? Remember, even if you can't share your private pains, just spending time with someone can be a valuable distraction and a meaningful part of your recovery.

### Getting Support for Your PPD

Look back where you listed people you could talk to about general things. Think carefully about these people. Isn't there one person on that list with whom you can talk about what you are going through? Would showing that person the introduction to this book help break the ice and get you started? We have heard from readers that sharing this book may help friends and family members learn more about PPD and how they can be more supportive to you.

Even the most well-meaning friends and family may say things that hurt, so it is critical to choose who you turn to for emotional support and to test the waters by starting small and working your way up only if you get some positive feedback. It is a very painful experience to risk telling someone that you have PPD, only to have that person shrug it off.

> Angie was talking to her best friend about how hurt she felt when her sister refused to take her PPD seriously. Right after Angie told her about it, her sister asked if she thought she would be "done with it" by next Sunday, when she needed Angie to watch the kids, because she had tickets to a basketball game. Her friend said: "You would think it's men who don't understand PPD—the truth is, it's the woman who had a perfect pregnancy, perfect delivery, and perfect baby who just doesn't have a clue."

Some people will make thoughtless, ridiculous, insulting, and un-informed comments if they find out that you have PPD, are in treat-ment, are taking medication, have been hospitalized, or even just don't feel as happy as they think you should. It may be helpful to know that you are not the only one who finds herself wondering about a sister-in-law who could say, "Do you think this happened because you wanted a boy?" or a friend who suggests that you are spoiled or whining. Hurtful comments are usually made out of lack of knowl-edge, not malice, and when you feel better, you may want to try to educate those who misunderstand PPD. Sometimes, the person comes around by herself. Angie's sister, for example, finally took her PPD seriously when she overheard a conversation in which her parents were talking to Angie's husband about how the three of them would manage to take care of the baby if Angie needed hospitalization. She suddenly realized the magnitude of Angie's illness and became much more supportive.

If there simply isn't anyone in your family or circle of friends who can be supportive about your illness, we urge you to find support online (PostpartumProgress.com or Postpartum.net) or find a support group for new mothers. This is often helpful even when you have a strong support network. There are now endless sources of online support through Facebook, Twitter, blogs, and long-standing websites like BabyCenter.com and ParentsPlace.com, just to name a couple. The Internet has proven to be a reliable way to "meet" other mothers who may be feeling the same way you are, but be careful selecting your support resources. The Internet is also full of way too much information, and it can be difficult to sift through it if you are having symptoms of anxiety or depression. Remember, not everything you read is true! Be sure to get your information and support from reputable websites.

Parents, siblings, in-laws, friends, and even helpful strangers can provide a significant amount of much-needed nurturing and strength. Indulge in it for a while. Let someone else take care of you for a change. Some women have problems getting relatives to help out more, while others have problems getting overprotective family members to do less, or to stand back once you begin to recover. The conflict around these issues may be lessened by 1) listening to yourself about what you need, 2) giving yourself permission to be nurtured, and 3) talking openly with your family about how they can help you most effectively.

And, of course, your greatest source of aid and encouragement will probably be your husband. In the next chapter, we discuss ways to enhance the support you get from your relationship with him.

# 9

# "What's Happening to My Marriage?"

## *Helping Your Husband to Help You*[*]

*John is trying to be supportive and do all the right things, but he
just doesn't understand what I'm going through. Sometimes I feel so
guilty about putting him through this, and then other times I wonder
why he can't help out more. Why do I have to explain what I need
from him over and over again? So I feel guilty, then I feel angry. I feel
him slipping farther away from me. I'm afraid our marriage can't
take this pressure—if he left now, I don't know what I'd do.*

—HEIDI, **PPD** SUPPORT-GROUP PARTICIPANT

*W*HAT CAN YOU DO to make it through what may be one of the
darkest phases in your marriage? Concern about the devastating impact that PPD may have on a marriage is prevalent and well-founded.

---

[*] It's worth repeating that throughout this book, we use the term *husband* to describe
your partner. We recognize that there are many ways in which families are constituted,
and that single, cohabiting, separated, or lesbian women are not immune to PPD. We use
*husband* because the majority of partners will be husbands.

Simply having a baby (whether it's the first or the third or fourth) is an enormously stressful event for couples. Several studies of new parents show that marital conflict and dissatisfaction are very common in the first year after childbirth. It may help to know that some of what you are feeling is due to the pressure every couple with a new baby feels, and it will get better. Unfortunately, your marriage has the extra burden of PPD. The stress on a marriage affected by PPD is like other aspects of "ordinary" postpartum stress—similar in kind to what other new parents experience, yet greatly intensified. It's no wonder you both feel so frustrated.

In Chapter 8, we asked you to assess your need for more support from friends and family. Here, we would like you to look at your need for more support from your husband. This is a critical part of your recovery, because research has shown that support from your husband can significantly reduce the severity and duration of the depression.

Consider the following questions and check those that apply to you:

_____ 1. Sometimes my husband seems distant and emotionally unavailable.

_____ 2. It is hard to divide my attention and love between my child and my husband.

_____ 3. I feel like I'm nagging every time I ask my husband to do one little thing.

_____ 4. My husband is happy to take care of the baby—it's me who never gets any of his affection.

_____ 5. I think he must be sorry he ever met me.

_____ 6. We never talk about the things that are wrong: our sex life, the fact that we have no money anymore, or the fact that we can't go ten minutes without an argument.

_____ 7. I know he's trying to be understanding—it's just that he never says the right thing.

Regardless of how strong their marriages are, we expect that the majority of readers will check at least one box. Occasionally, women with PPD report that their relationship and lines of communication with their husbands are unaffected by PPD. Most husbands will try to support you as you cope with PPD, both in the short and long term. However, some may never understand PPD; others are sympathetic at first but lose patience after a while. Sometimes, husbands are worse than unsupportive: they may say things that hurt you, seem to blame you for your illness, or become abusive. But even when your husband is trying his best, you may find that nothing he says or does feels like enough.

Before you continue on to learn how to get more support from your husband, it may be helpful to put yourself in his shoes for a moment and consider some of the pressures he's feeling. He may be emotionally preoccupied with his own issues or insecurities as he works through this major life transition. Just as our attitudes and ideas about mothering are changing, so is our vision of fatherhood. We now expect men to be very involved in the care of a new baby, as the media flood us with images of loving, diaper-changing, nurturing dads. At the same time, very few men have either role models for this kind of involvement or support at the workplace for making fathering a priority. Husbands need validation, too—a simple acknowledgment or a thank-you for his efforts can go a long way. When you have PPD, the experience of day-to-day living is often so overwhelming that bolstering him seems almost impossible, but it is important to try.

You may wish to read Chapter 10, which addresses your husband's needs in greater depth. For now, we will focus on what you need from the relationship, and how to increase the likelihood of receiving it.

## Effective Communication: A Primer

Long before a baby is born, most couples have developed habitual ways of oblique communication. For example, many couples have nonverbal ways of communicating sexual overtures: a back rub is recognized by both members as an invitation for making love. Similarly, they may have personally coded ways of requesting reassurance: "Does this dress look okay?" is recognized as "Do you still find me attractive? Are you still glad you married me?" The trash bag by the back door may be mutually understood as "Please take the trash out on your way to the car."

Indirect communication can be effective when things are going smoothly. However, the stress that PPD places on your marriage requires you to develop new ways of relating to each other and to actively strengthen clear and direct communication. In our practices, we often help both husband and wife to understand each other's views and needs, because repetitive misunderstandings can lead to chronic resentments that will drive a stressed-out couple even farther apart. One such couple is Ted and Maria:

Maria was fed up with Ted. He never offered to do one thing for the baby, and he didn't seem to appreciate how hard it was for her to "just stay home." His preoccupation with problems at work seemed petty in comparison to her struggles to care for this needy, fragile person when she felt so vulnerable herself. And then there was The Look: the disapproval she read in his expression when he walked in the door at 6 p.m. and saw that the pile of clothes she meant to take to the laundromat was still sitting by the front door. He seemed so self-absorbed—did she have to remind him to be quiet every time the baby was sleeping? She knew he was having a hard time at work, so she didn't want to criticize him, but enough is enough. . . .

Ted was fed up with Maria. She seemed obsessed with the baby— it was as if she wished he would just go away and leave the two of them alone. When he offered to do something as simple as laundry, she complained that he used the wrong detergent or didn't fold it right, so he quit asking. Even when the baby went to sleep, she only wanted to talk about the trivialities of how many ounces of formula the baby took or whether she should consult the doctor about the tiny pimple she noticed on the baby's forehead that day. She certainly wasn't interested in hearing about his work. He knew she was having a hard time with anxiety attacks, so he didn't want to criticize her, but enough is enough.

In the upheaval of this major change in their lives, both Ted and Maria are misinterpreting each other's feelings, behaviors, and attitudes. Each perceives the other as being uninterested in the other's daily activities—Ted feels Maria doesn't care about his problems at work, while Maria feels Ted doesn't care about her problems at home. Each tries to engage the other's interest by talking more and more about the details of the day, but this is misunderstood as proof that the other is self-absorbed. Hurt and angry feelings smoulder, and the miscommunication begins to take on a life of its own. The only way to bridge the growing divide is through direct communication.

Many women have been conditioned to avoid direct expression of their needs, because not so long ago it was considered selfish or "unladylike" to draw attention to themselves or their requirements. They may find it very difficult or embarrassing to ask for support, and many even fear that asking for too much will drive their husbands away. Before we go any farther, let us reassure you: your needs are only human and are nothing to be ashamed of; you are entitled to ask for and receive support from those around you. Of course, certain approaches to asking for support are more successful than others, and the manner in which you ask can do a lot to keep you from sounding like a nag or a whiner.

Consider the most common ways women express their needs for support to their husbands: "I need your support." One of the reasons this may not stimulate the reaction you want from your husband is that it's too general and vague. "I need your support" can be more effectively expressed by addressing specific behaviors or actions to be taken. For example: "I would feel better if you called your family and told them we can't make it tonight. I'm not feeling up to it," or

"Could you please put the kids to bed tonight so I can have a break?" or "I need a hug right now!"

Often, women preface their pleas for support by saying, "You know I'm feeling sad. Why can't you help with . . . " This approach often backfires, because it sounds as if you expect your husband to be a mind reader. The same request is more effectively communicated by the following: "I'm feeling especially sad right now. This is so hard for me. Can you help me with the . . . " Here you avoid implying that your husband should know exactly how you feel at all times and should act accordingly. Accusatory comments such as "Why are you coming home so late, when I'm so overwhelmed?" immediately make him feel guilty and defensive, and may cause him to take the offensive in order to defend himself. The conflict rapidly escalates, and the request for help is lost in an argument over who is more overwhelmed. Try instead, "The days are long for me now. I would feel better if I could look forward to a break when you got home. Maybe you can work it out so that you were home earlier some of the time."

In sum, keep these points in mind when communicating your needs:

- Never assume your husband knows how you are feeling at any time.
- Be very specific about what you need at this time.
- State your needs in terms of what you need and feel, not in terms of what he's doing or not doing.

Additional Communication Tips:

**Use "I" statements, rather than "you" statements:**
For example: I feel so alone when you spend all evening in
  the den.
*instead of*
You never spend time with me.

**Try an empathic statement in which you acknowledge his position first, then your desire:**

For example: I know you're tired from work, but I could use some advice about . . . I see you're busy, but when you have a free moment I'd like to talk.

instead of

You're finally home! What do you want to do about . . .

**Test the waters before making a direct statement:**

For example: I would like to spend an evening alone with you. How do you feel about going out for a bite to eat tonight?

instead of

I'm not cooking again tonight!

**Don't be afraid to make a direct request:**

For example: Please answer the phone if it rings. Please reassure me that I'm doing a good job.

instead of

I hate that phone. I feel like such a failure.

## Helping Him to Help You

Categorizing your need for support from your husband will help you develop ways to meet these specific needs. We encourage you to look at your relationship with your husband from the following perspectives: practical support, emotional needs, and sexuality issues in PPD.

Again, let us reassure you that every woman with PPD is likely to have some need for more support from her husband in each of these three areas.

### PRACTICAL SUPPORT

As we discussed in the last chapter, getting support in concrete, practical ways can provide some of the physical and emotional breathing room you need to begin to take care of yourself. For some women, this is the easiest place to begin asking for help; for other women, it is the most difficult. Many husbands are eager to provide practical, hands-on assistance. They want to do something, and having an explicit task "assigned" to them helps them feel more involved in your recovery.

Consider some of the practical ways that your husband can provide support.

He can . . .

- pick up the dry cleaning
- answer the phone and say you're sleeping
- do the laundry or other housework
- make dinner, order in, or pick up take-out food on the way home from work
- ask his mother or sister to come over and be with you during some of the time he's at work
- drive you to your doctor's appointment
- take responsibility for the baby's bath, diaper changing, or nighttime bottles when he's around

Can you think of any other examples? Once you've come up with some of the ways your husband can offer hands-on help, the next step is to ask for it. If this is hard for you, go back to the previous section and try to match one specific need with one of the communication tips offered and mentally rehearse your statement. For example, match a request to pick up your prescription with an acknowledgment of his position: "I know your day is long already, but it would really help me out if you could swing by the pharmacy on your way home to get my new prescription. They told me it would be ready, so you won't have to wait." Keep practicing this—eventually it will feel more natural.

Like Maria, some wives expect their husbands to do a certain task exactly the way they would do it. This way of thinking can backfire, though. Ted pulled back even farther when Maria corrected how he folded the laundry. Just as you don't have to do everything perfectly, neither does your husband. Ignore the flaws in how he helps you out and let him figure out his own way of doing things—he'll feel better about providing this kind of support, and you will get more help.

## EMOTIONAL NEEDS

"Couple time" is typically the first thing given up in order to make room for the enormous demands the baby makes on your time. Many women describe an almost reflexive effort to "put the relationship on hold" for a while and report that they hardly miss it until the pain of isolation or tension in the marriage becomes unbearable. In other words, in the effort to put all of your energy and most of your self into the care of the new baby, you may inadvertently be shutting out one of the most valuable resources you have to help you manage your new responsibilities.

During periods of severe stress, feelings get polarized into extremes: everything appears to be either black or white. When it comes to your feelings about your husband, at times you may feel so negatively toward him that you can't imagine that he could be compassionate and reassuring to you. Or you may feel so isolated from each other that it is difficult to look forward to ever feeling as close as you once did. If you feel cut off from him emotionally, it will be especially difficult—but also especially important—to ask for this kind of support.

Often, the feeling of being abandoned emotionally stems from a disappointment in his inability to intuit what you need. "Why do I have to spell everything out?" is a complaint that we often hear. At a deep level, you may believe that if he *really* loved you, you wouldn't have to ask him for support—he would just know what to do. One woman in treatment said, "I know it's irrational, but I want him to act like a perfect mother—to know what I need from him *before* I'm even conscious of it."

While it is perfectly natural to wish for the romantic ideal of a man who instinctively knows what you need, it is not fair (and is often self-defeating) to expect that of your flesh-and-blood husband. Instead, you must accept that you have to articulate what emotional support you need and how he can provide it for you. No matter how much your husband may love you or how close your relationship is, your husband cannot read your mind.

Be as specific about your emotional needs as you were about your need for hands-on help. Just as your husband will not know that you would like him to go to the dry cleaners unless you ask, he will not be able to make the jump from "I need more emotional support" to understanding that you need him to let you know that he thinks you are doing a good job taking care of your baby. This may seem very simple, but it's true. The only way he can know what you need is for you to know what you need and for you to communicate that to him somehow. When Maria finally told Ted directly that she was terrified of missing something physically wrong with the baby, he stopped rolling his eyes when she obsessed about every little blotch on the baby. He really helped her by saying, "We're both new at this, so I'm sure we're bound to make mistakes. But I can't imagine that you wouldn't notice anything serious."

The following exercise is designed to help you assess your own emotional needs:

1. I wish my husband would do *more* of the following:
Example: Sit next to me and hold my hand, so I don't feel so alone.
a) _____
b) _____
2. I wish my husband would do *less* of the following:
   Example: Trying to do something to "fix" this PPD, instead of accepting it and helping me live with the illness for now.
a) _____
b) _____

3. He just doesn't seem to understand that, sometimes, all I need is:

_____

_____

4. When I'm feeling sad, I like him to:

_____

_____

5. I think the most important thing I want him to know right now is:

_____

_____

6. Sometimes, I'm afraid to tell him how I really feel, because:

_____

_____

As you did in the section on practical support, try linking one specific emotional need with a communication tip. When it comes to expressing emotional needs, "I" statements are often especially helpful. For example, if you want him to complain less about how much your therapy is costing, try a statement such as, "When I hear you make jokes about how expensive my therapy is, I feel so guilty. I feel bad about how much it costs, too."

It is also particularly important to remember to let him know when he does or says something that makes you feel good. He can't read your mind, so you need to reassure him that you do notice and appreciate his efforts.

## Talking About Sex

While sexuality is generally the hardest issue for women with PPD to talk about with their husbands, it is almost always a concern:

By the time my husband would come home at 7:30, I was exhausted from getting the boys ready for bed and cleaning up after dinner. I could feel the pressure building up inside me—I felt like I would explode if he touched me at all.

I guess he got the message, because we don't talk about it anymore, and he never touches me. Frankly, I feel relieved, but of course I feel guilty about that. I swear if he came home and said we would never have sex again, I would be thrilled.

Many women temporarily lose interest in sex after the birth of a child, whether or not they suffer from PPD. A variety of factors affect your sexuality at this time. Depending on how many months postpartum you are and your own psychology, some of these may have a greater impact than others.

Episiotomy stitches, caesarian-section recovery, breastfeeding (leakage, tenderness, self-consciousness, and hormone changes), exhaustion, vaginal dryness due to temporary hormone changes, and a fear of getting pregnant again all may contribute to postpartum loss of sex drive. Women with PPD also often suffer from profound fatigue, low self-esteem, poor body image, and biochemical changes in the part of the brain that regulates sexuality. Many clinicians see loss of sex drive as a hallmark of depression.

When you have PPD, you are very vulnerable to feeling shame and guilt, and it is harder to shake feelings of inadequacy. As you look over these factors, can you allow yourself to feel less guilty about your loss of sexual interest? This is important, because shame interferes with communicating about sexuality. You need to accept the sexual self you are right now, as the first step to letting your husband know what you need.

Sexual tension is almost always present in couples affected by PPD. It helps to conceptualize this tension as a mismatch. At times that you may be feeling a decrease in your sexual interest, your husband may be feeling the exact opposite. He may find your changing body very attractive, may be exhilarated by the potency of fathering a child, or may be eager to resume an active physical relationship that has been put on hold by childbearing. The fact that his sexual drive and your lack of sexual drive are out of synch doesn't mean that your sexual relationship is gone for good.

Talking about sexuality is extremely difficult for most couples, even when everything else is going well. Many feel this is a part of their relationship that should take care of itself naturally, as long as the love, intimacy, and commitment are intact. But this is not the case.

If having sex is not on your agenda right now, talking about it must be. This first step is the best way to avoid the misunderstandings that can lead to anger and hurt feelings later. If you find it is too embarrassing to talk about sex face-to-face, try talking about it on the phone or in the car (when you both are looking forward and don't have to face each other). As a last resort, leave him a note asking him to talk with you about this. A therapist can also be very helpful in helping you overcome the initial embarrassment.

Miscommunication frequently arises because women with PPD and the low sex drive associated with it also often have an increased need for affection and touching. Some women hesitate to pursue this need, because they are afraid that their husbands will interpret a reassuring cuddle as an overture for making love. They may feel hurt or angry if their husbands do indeed become aroused by touching, leaving the men confused by what seems like a mixed nonverbal message. Intimacy suffers when couples can't talk about what they really want.

Once Maria mastered learning to ask Ted directly for practical and emotional support, she took a deep breath and tackled their sexual relationship. One night, they were watching television from separate places in the living room. She said, "It would feel so good to have you come lie next to me on the couch and hold me. I don't have any sex drive still, but I really miss being physically close with you."

Ted immediately joined Maria on the couch and gave her a back rub. She could tell by his breathing that he did get aroused, but he didn't push, and she didn't feel guilty. The next morning, he spent a few extra minutes stroking her hair before he got out of bed.

We encourage you to maintain or reestablish simple touching. This land of nonsexual touching is a vital part of your relationship with your husband. With all of the changes going on right now, what you need is some consistent, nonthreatening expressions of affection, security, and trust. Sometimes a touch can do just that—but you need to ask.

You can say:

- Can you spare five minutes for a foot rub? I think it might help me fall asleep, and I know it would feel great.
- My doctor told me to tell you that my sex drive will return when I recover. She says if it doesn't, I can adjust my medication and that should help.
- I hope you don't take this personally. It's me, not you. I miss our sex life, too, but I just don't have any interest in making love right now. I do really like to hold hands and hug, and hope you do, too.
- I feel guilty about never wanting to make love. I really appreciate how understanding you've been about it.

It may still be tempting to try to place your relationship with your husband on hold until you recover from PPD. To do so robs you of an opportunity to use the experience of PPD to actually strengthen your bond. Those couples who have reached a deeper level of communication and caring by going through PPD together will leave the experience of PPD with that much more strength to face life's other challenges together.

The next chapter is written for your husband, although you may find it interesting to read as well. The same issues we have covered for

you in this chapter will be discussed from his point of view. By raising these issues with both of you, we hope that those of you who are
stuck in patterns of hurt feelings and miscommunication will open
new avenues of discussion. Those couples who are managing successfully may also find some useful tips to further communication.

PPD can test a marriage like nothing else you've ever encountered.
Embrace the challenge, and you may find your marriage emerges
with new vitality and endurance.

# 10

# "WILL MY WIFE EVER BE THE SAME?"

## When Your Wife Has Postpartum Depression

*I don't understand this. We waited for this baby for so long. We
planned for it and dreamed about this time together. Everything
seemed to be falling into place. Now, all of a sudden, nothing
makes sense. I've never seen her act this way. I've never seen her
give up like this—she used to be so strong. She isn't doing the
things she used to—she's just crying all the time and says she
can't help it. I don't know what the hell is going on anymore.*

—PAUL, WHOSE WIFE HAS PPD

*W*HAT'S GOING ON is that your wife is suffering from postpartum depression or anxiety (we refer to this as "PPD" for
the rest of the chapter), a condition that afflicts many women after
childbirth. Your interest in learning about PPD is a tremendous asset
for your wife as well as for you. She is struggling to overcome this illness, but she needs your help, too. This chapter will help you translate
your interest and energy into positive steps that will help her recover.

The most important step is understanding that PPD is an illness that really does exist. Your wife is not making it up, and she is not going crazy. It is not easy to define PPD, and you are probably searching for a very concise explanation: What is it? Where did it come from? How do we get our lives back to normal as soon as possible? Along with the questions, you may share the fears that Jim has about his wife Michelle:

> Jim's first response to Michelle's PPD was anger. He was angry at her for being so needy, angry at the obstetrician for not warning them, angry at Michelle's family for not helping out more, and angry that out of all the new fathers he knew, he was the only one who wasn't thoroughly enjoying this new phase of life.
>
> Gradually, Jim's anger was replaced by fear. As Michelle became more and more withdrawn, as the panicky phone calls at work escalated, he worried that the Michelle he married was gone for good. He was afraid that she'd live her whole life as a shell of her past. When she sought professional help, he worried that she would be "hooked" on her medications, or spend the next five years dependent on her therapist. Although he could see that Michelle was perfectly able to care for their daughter, he couldn't get the stories of mothers who killed their babies out of his head, and he secretly worried that the doctor was wrong when she said that Michelle wouldn't hurt their baby.

Unfortunately, psychiatric illness is so stigmatized that, like Jim, most people know nothing at all about it until a family member is afflicted. In the absence of facts, all the myths, distortions, and deep fears rush in to fill the gap. For centuries, psychiatric illness was a life sentence: confinement and loss of function were common, because there were not effective treatments. But in the last several decades, psychiatric knowledge has increased exponentially, and new information about how the brain works, along with highly specialized medications and talk therapies, have made full recovery from depression and anxiety a reality. We believe that in the near future, psychiatric illness will no longer be stigmatized, but will be viewed in the same way we view physical sickness.

Depression and anxiety after childbirth are real illnesses with excellent prognoses. Most experts believe that PPD results from a combination of physiological, biochemical, hormonal, psychological, and social factors that affect a woman after the birth of a baby. Depending on your wife's particular circumstances, these factors interacted in such a way as to give her PPD. We do not fully understand why PPD afflicts some women and not others. But we do know that it is neither your fault nor hers that she has PPD. It did not occur because of something you or she felt, thought, did, or feared.

PPD has a characteristic set of symptoms, including changes in emotions, behaviors, and sleep and eating patterns. If your wife has PPD, you may notice that she is inclined to:

- Feel sad and worthless
- Have sleeping difficulties
- Eat less or more
- Withdraw from friends
- Cry excessively
- Feel tired
- Lose interest in activities
- Lose sexual desire
- Be very irritable
- Have physical complaints
- Have anxiety attacks, or feel anxious all the time
- Feel guilty
- Feel inadequate
- Feel angry
- Criticize you frequently
- Fail to notice your efforts
- Fail to respond to reassurance

Unfortunately, when PPD occurs, it is most often the husband who is left carrying much of the load. Depending on the severity of your wife's depression or anxiety, the burden of caring for the baby, the house, and your wife, along with your job and other ongoing responsibilities, may become overwhelming.

The first part of this chapter will provide specific suggestions that will help you help your wife. The next part of the chapter will address your needs and how you can best help yourself through this. We end with a true story of a physician's experience with his wife's PPD.

## What You Can Do for Her

Some of the basic ways of helping your wife through this period may be so straightforward as to appear trivial to you. But you'd be surprised—in her heightened state of isolation and insecurity, how just hearing you express your concern or make a simple offer to run an errand can bring her untold peace of mind. Unfortunately, sometimes PPD is so severe that you can't seem to do anything right. Even when this is the case, your attempts to help her are registering subconsciously—when she recovers, she will be able to appreciate all your efforts.

Here are some specific ways that you can help your wife.

### LISTEN AND VALIDATE

Let her tell you how she's feeling, even if she's telling you the same thing over and over again. She doesn't think this will ever get better. But trust us, it will get better. Listen to her. Let her know you believe her and you will be there for her no matter what. She is very aware of the extra burden you are carrying, and one of her greatest fears is that you will get tired of this and abandon her.

Your wife's conviction that her pain won't get better is actually a symptom of this illness. PPD robs a woman of the ability to envision future happiness. This makes it important not to say, "Stop worrying so much—you'll get over it." Instead, you might say, "I know it seems that you will always feel this way. I also know that Dr. Smith is certain that you will get back to your old self."

Your instincts about what to do may not work, or may actually increase the emotional distance between the two of you. For example, responding to her distress with logic or advice, or trying to be firm with her, may not be effective, because they may make her feel misunderstood or alienated from you. Although your first response may be total disbelief, saying things like, "What's wrong with you?" or "Snap out of it!" will not make her feel better. This is new territory for you both, and you cannot expect yourself to know how to comfort her intuitively. Knowing what to do—and what not to do—is not a sign of how much you love your wife. If you find that you can't seem to do anything to help, don't be afraid to ask her therapist, her doctor, or someone else who has gone through this for advice.

Pitfalls to avoid include:

* Pretending it isn't happening
* Criticizing or judging her
* Blaming her or someone else for the PPD
* Smothering her or overreacting
* Becoming overly preoccupied with why she is feeling what she is feeling instead of just accepting her feelings

## TRY TO BE PATIENT

We know how much you want things to return to "normal" so you can get on with your life. After so much anticipation and excitement around the birth of your baby, this is devastating. But wishing things back to normal will not make them so.

Recovery from PPD is usually gradual; at its worst, each day can seem like an eternity. Knowing this can help you pace yourself and keep you from expecting things to change dramatically overnight. You might also have to help your wife to be patient, as this is often one of the most difficult aspects of PPD for her to come to terms with, as well. We see many fathers who, once the PPD is identified, feel compelled to "fix" it. It is perfectly understandable that you both want this to go away immediately. Unfortunately, there are no quick fixes or magic spells to ease the pain.

It will be helpful to remind her that PPD does get better, even though it takes some time. Try to be specific when reassuring her. For example, remind yourselves that the doctor said that antidepressants may take a month or more before an effect is seen, that her therapist warned you that some symptoms may linger for months, or that a bad day doesn't necessarily mean she's getting worse.

## PROVIDE BREAKS FOR YOUR WIFE

Whenever possible, squeeze in some extra breaks for her so she can rest, relax, or indulge in some pleasure. Ask her what you can do for her, what would help her feel a little better. Help her be specific about what she wants or what you can do to free her up a bit. Like David, you may not be able to assume that she will ask for help:

Due to a special project at the office, David had been working seven days a week. As soon as the project was done, he offered to take the baby to the park on a Saturday morning. He told his wife, Naomi, "I want you to take a bubble bath, take a nap, do whatever makes you happy. I forbid you to do *any* housework while we're out. So what if the house isn't perfect—you need a break, too!"

His wife burst out crying. At first he thought he had somehow hurt her feelings, but she explained that she was crying because she was so touched by his offer. She thought, "I was sure he hadn't noticed how hard things have been for me at home." He thought, "I had no idea that she'd been under such pressure that she thought she needed my permission to take a break. Does she think I care more about the house than I do about her?"

David realized that he needed to make regular offers of assistance: Should he pick up dinner on the way home? Was there a load of laundry he could do for her at night? Could he call his sister to see if she could watch the baby while she got a haircut? Would she meet him downtown for lunch one day? Could they go for a walk together after he got home? Was there anything they needed from the grocery store?

Suggest that your wife exercise and get out of the house more, but remember that this may be very difficult for someone who is depressed, and she may be particularly sensitive about her body right now. You should encourage but not push. If you can afford it, give her specific permission to hire temporary assistance, such as a babysitter, mother's helper, or occasional housecleaner, or to buy more convenience foods or order pizza for dinner once in a while.

### GIVE HER PERMISSION TO BE LESS INTERESTED IN SEX

Most women with PPD will not be interested in sex. Your wife's sexual interest and energy will return when she begins to feel more like herself. It is important that you not take this personally. Reassure her that this is okay and that you won't cheat on her or leave her because she doesn't want to have sex with you right now. While suffering from PPD, your wife may be more interested in touching or holding that does not lead to sex. Many women feel an increased need to be held and comforted during this time. They may be afraid to express this need, either verbally or physically, because they don't want to "mislead" you into thinking they may be interested in making love. Talk to her about this. Let her tell you exactly how she feels about being touched right now.

### PROVIDE EMOTIONAL SUPPORT

Because your wife may be in a state of heightened sensitivity, it may be difficult to figure out what to say to be supportive. Try the following:

- Tell her you love her.
- Notice and comment appreciatively on small achievements, such as getting out thank-you notes, or doing a household task that she couldn't do before. Back off immediately if she perceives this as condescending.
- Reassure your wife that you don't regret marrying her.
- Let her know that you are glad that she is the mother of your child.
- Be especially sensitive to how your wife feels about her body right now. Notice if her hair looks nice, or if she is wearing a pretty outfit. Tell her you think she's pretty.
- Remind her that you will stick by her side, just as she would if you were sick.

## SUPPORT HER DECISION TO SEEK HELP

It is important for you to support her decision to seek help, whether through individual therapy, medication, support groups, workshops, play groups, or elsewhere. It is always a plus if you can participate. Any decision she is able to make at this time should be encouraged (as long as it is safe—more about this shortly).

If your wife is currently in therapy, show an interest in her progress. Going to a therapy session with her can be beneficial for three reasons: 1) it shows support, 2) it will help clarify the picture for you, and you can have some of your own questions answered directly, and 3) your presence will help provide new and valuable information to her therapist for further evaluation and treatment.

Many husbands find it extremely helpful to participate in the decision about whether their wives should take medication for PPD, although the final decision must be left up to her. A visit with her psychiatrist may answer many questions for you or help you to help her make the best decision. If you are unfamiliar with psychiatric medications, or if you are totally opposed to this treatment option, it is important that you read Chapter 6, which discusses the option of medication. Since this may be a critical part of your wife's recovery, it is essential to remain objective and open-minded. If it is suggested that she give up breastfeeding in order to take medication, let her know that her health is very important to you and that you still consider her to be a good mother.

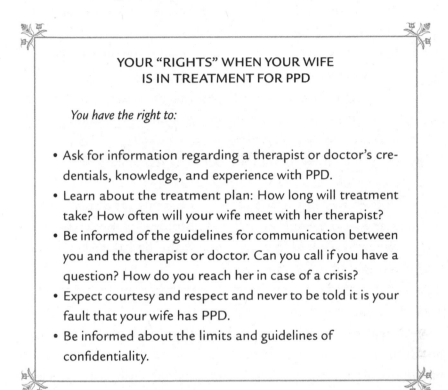

### YOUR "RIGHTS" WHEN YOUR WIFE IS IN TREATMENT FOR PPD

*You have the right to:*

- Ask for information regarding a therapist or doctor's credentials, knowledge, and experience with PPD.
- Learn about the treatment plan: How long will treatment take? How often will your wife meet with her therapist?
- Be informed of the guidelines for communication between you and the therapist or doctor. Can you call if you have a question? How do you reach her in case of a crisis?
- Expect courtesy and respect and never to be told it is your fault that your wife has PPD.
- Be informed about the limits and guidelines of confidentiality.

Remember that you are a very integral part of your wife's treatment, and your support can make a big difference in how quickly she will recover. Your wife may feel extremely guilty about the cost of treatment, and may even claim she doesn't want professional help because she is afraid of imposing a financial burden on the family. Reassure her that her health is of paramount importance and that you will find a way to handle the bills. If possible, avoid dwelling on the cost of treatment. Some options you may want to investigate include:

- Negotiate a payment plan on her behalf.
- Confirm the details of your insurance coverage. Get the specifics of the copayment, the maximum fee per session, which types of professionals are covered, and whether there is a maximum number of sessions or total coverage per calendar year. Clarify the difference between her inpatient and outpatient mental-health benefits.
- Look into centers or agencies with sliding-scale fees. These include mental-health centers and training programs, such as a nearby medical school's psychiatry residency program, or a university graduate school program in psychology or social work, as well as some private clinical practices.
- Don't be afraid to ask the doctor or therapist if she or he has a policy for financial hardship.
- Consider asking your and/or her parents for a small loan. Many new parents turn to grandparents for unexpected expenses associated with a new baby, and this should be thought of in the same way.

Some men find it hard to support their wives' decision to seek professional treatment, because deep down inside they feel that a good husband should be able to "fix" any problem. For some husbands, a male therapist or psychiatrist may be intimidating, because they feel criticized or inept when another man tells them how to treat their own wives. Your wife doesn't need treatment because you have failed! If she broke her leg, you wouldn't feel guilty because a doctor needed to set it.

Some men are in the opposite situation: he desperately wants her to seek treatment, but she refuses. In most cases, she is making a faulty decision (often because the PPD itself causes her to believe that nothing will help), but not a dangerous one. If treatment is not an emergency, you may be able to compromise on a time when she will agree to treatment. For example, you might agree that if she is not better in two weeks, she will obtain a professional consultation. Then you must give her a chance to try to do it her way for whatever period of time you agree upon.

## MONITOR FOR SIGNS OF AN EMERGENCY

Note: If you do not have any concerns about the possibility that your wife might hurt herself or the baby, skip the next section and go to "What you can do for yourself."

If you think that your wife or the baby is in danger, you must override her decision to avoid treatment. Someone who is at risk of hurting herself or hurting someone else can be legally forced to receive treatment and/or hospitalization. Again, this is very scary but also very rare. Danger signs to watch for include the following:

- Talk of hurting herself or your baby
- Bizarre thinking patterns, hallucinations, delusions
- Withdrawal from all social contact
- Expressions like, "You would be better off without me" or "I just wish I could sleep and never wake up"
- Preoccupation with death or morbid ideas
- Extreme, persistent feelings of hopelessness
- Increased risk-taking behaviors or self-destructive behaviors

There is a myth that people who talk about suicide don't actually do it. The opposite is true: any hints or open discussion of self-harm must be taken very seriously. If you think she may be suicidal, listen carefully, and do not ignore or minimize what she says. Make sure you have emergency phone numbers posted near your phones (doctor, therapist, ambulance, etc.). Or you can call 911 (or the emergency police number if you don't have 911) for immediate assistance, or take her to any emergency room twenty-four hours a day. **DO NOT LEAVE HER ALONE FOR ANY REASON**. Initiate child care alternatives and monitor all medication until she is out of danger.

## What You Can Do for Yourself

Remembering to take care of yourself right now is every bit as important as taking care of your wife. Undoubtedly, your expectations about what the first few months of new fatherhood would be like were very different from the reality of PPD. Like many men whose wives have PPD, you may be subject to unwelcome or painful comments from coworkers, relatives, and friends. Burnout is a real risk—here are steps you can take to avoid exhaustion.

### GIVE YOURSELF CREDIT

First of all, recognize how tough this is for you. It is unreasonable to expect yourself to know what to do or to be able to manage everything all the time. The first few months after childbirth are stressful for new fathers, even when things go as smoothly as possible. When you add having a wife with PPD, the first months can be the worst time of life that you have ever experienced. There is far more support built into our society for a new mother than there is for a new father.

Most men whose wives have PPD face all the pressures of continuing to work while simultaneously doing more of the household and child care responsibilities than was anticipated, all the while being chronically sleep deprived. Many men find that having a child precipitates an increased sense of urgency about providing for the family's financial well-being. At the same time, if your wife calls you at work several times a day or asks you to come home early on a regular basis, you may feel that her PPD is in conflict with your ability to work. No wonder you feel pulled in all directions! Give yourself a pat on the back before you do anything else, because it may be a while before anyone else recognizes what a wonderful job you are doing.

### TALK ABOUT THIS WITH SOMEONE YOU TRUST

It is very important for you to find someone to discuss the situation with, as talking is absolutely the most underrated way to manage this emotional assault. Seek out close friends, relatives, or other young fathers—you may be surprised how many others have wives who suffered from PPD. Ask how they coped and consider trying to do what worked for them. Occasionally, a new-fathers' support group is available; a few sessions with a professional therapist may also be very helpful.

Some men say that they have a difficult time expressing their feelings to other men, because issues related to how men are raised, male role expectations, and self-identity get in the way. In this case, consider talking to your sister or your mother or your wife's close friend. Alternatively, this may be an opportunity for you to take some risks of your own—you may discover a new level of support you hadn't realized was available from your men friends.

After David canceled the third racquetball game in a row, his friend Phil started teasing him: "What's wrong, wife got you changing so many diapers you can't even take an hour off?"

David said, "If you only knew!"

Immediately, Phil got serious. "What do you mean? Is something wrong between the two of you?"

David tested the waters: "Did you ever hear of postpartum depression?"

Phil surprised him: "Sure, my wife's sister had that. My brother-in-law was a wreck, too."

They didn't say much more, but it cleared the air for them both. Phil understood that David wasn't avoiding him, and David felt relieved to unburden his secret. Phil's last words were music to his ears: "You know, my sister-in-law is fine now. You'd never know it even happened."

Although it may be tempting to go it alone, talking about how you feel to someone you trust will help you get perspective on your feelings and reactions. You might be surprised how good it can feel.

## TAKE GOOD CARE OF YOURSELF

We know it sounds too simple to be true, but it really is important for you to take care of yourself. You need to eat well, sleep well, exercise, and rest whenever possible (not easy, we know). All of these things will combine to fortify your resources at a time when you need them the most. The risk of not taking care of yourself can be high. It might surprise you to learn that a recent study determined that up to 14 percent of fathers in the United States experience depression after the birth of their child. Men who have a history of depression are at highest risk. If you are concerned about the way you are feeling, be sure to let someone know.

If you are not exercising on a regular basis, you may discover that adding that to your routine will not only help you feel better physically, but will also provide an invaluable outlet for much of your built-up tensions and anxieties. Consider hiring a teenager to come over on a Saturday morning to watch the baby for an hour or two, so that you can go work out. Or you might want to invest in an infant bike carrier or a jogging stroller, so that you can exercise without feeling guilty about leaving your wife with the baby.

Don't forget to do something fun for yourself, too. Sometimes, you are so busy working, taking care of the baby, or doing something nice for your wife, that you forget that you need some of those goodies, too. Stay in touch with friends. Have a friend over to watch a football game on Sunday—you can keep an eye on the baby, give your wife a break, and still enjoy yourself. Admit that you need some good stuff in your life right now.

## TRY NOT TO TAKE HER COMPLAINTS TOO PERSONALLY

During her depression, your wife is likely to become hypercritical. Some of her expectations may be unreasonable and demanding. She may totally misinterpret all of your good efforts and intentions. It's hard not to take all of this personally, but you must try to remember that a lot of this is her illness talking. For example, Jim's wife Michelle sometimes reacted to his offers to help as if he were patronizing her. If he noticed any slight improvement, she felt as if he wasn't taking her distress seriously. If he said and did nothing, she accused him of not caring. Only when she recovered did she let him know how much she appreciated all his support.

## GIVE YOURSELF PERMISSION TO HAVE
## NEGATIVE FEELINGS ABOUT THIS SITUATION

After you have waited for the birth of your baby with so much excitement and anticipation, the letdown of PPD can be devastating. Everyone expects this time of life to be full of love and contentment. It doesn't seem fair that, instead, you have a home filled with endless hours of unexplained sadness and confusion. At times, you may feel cheated or very angry. *It is important for you to know that it is okay to be angry at the situation or angry at your wife's PPD, without being angry directly at your wife.*

You may also be feeling fear right now that stems from your lack of control over your wife's illness. Feeling so powerless while someone you love is in so much distress can be extremely frightening.

These feelings of frustration, anger, and fear are perfectly understandable and reasonable. Negative feelings should not be avoided or denied; instead, they must be expressed in a constructive way. Sometimes, a husband expresses his anger directly at his wife or child. Sometimes, he may withdraw and make himself unavailable emotionally or physically. Other times, he may channel these feelings into areas where he feels more secure; for instance, work may become the focus for much of his emotional energy. When these patterns of behavior persist, the husband becomes exhausted, and the family becomes depleted.

Robert's wife Maddie was two months postpartum when she got PPD. Before that time, he had tried to be supportive, but he knew that he just couldn't keep it up. He was jealous that she got to take time off from work to be with their new baby and jealous that the baby got all her attention. He felt ashamed of these feelings, but he had to admit that he hadn't expected his wife to practically ignore him for weeks on end. Just when he thought their sex life was about to resume, she developed PPD, with severe anxiety attacks and a fear of leaving the house.

Robert couldn't seem to do anything right for her, so he decided to quit trying. He threw himself into his job, taking any overtime hours that were available, telling himself that they needed the extra money. Some nights, he'd get home at 11:00 p.m., crash, and have to be back at work by 7:00 the next morning. When four days went by without any type of conversation with Maddie, Robert turned to his brother for advice. He admitted to throwing himself into his work in order to avoid being home, but repeated how much they needed the extra money.

Robert's brother said to him, "It seems like you already know what you need to do," and Robert realized that he was right. The next day he came home by 8:00 p.m. His mother-in-law, who had moved in to help out, noticed his efforts even though it was a while before Maddie said anything.

If any of this sounds familiar to you, you are not alone. It is tempting to try to avoid all the strong negative feelings that PPD can bring up. We're conditioned by society to repress and sublimate negative feelings. But bottled up long enough, they can explode, so it's better to find a healthy way to release them. Knowledge and awareness of what is going on can help ease your frustration and fear. Until you can admit to having these uncomfortable feelings, you cannot move ahead to do what needs to be done to take care of yourself and to help your wife.

This is the only chapter in the book that is specifically for you and not your wife. However, you may find that other parts of this book are helpful. For example, you might want to read the first chapter in order to learn more about the types and causes of PPD. You might want to read about coping skills if your wife keeps asking you what she should do. You might want to read about the varieties of professional treatment that are available, or whatever other chapters seem particularly appropriate to your situation.

The examples we've provided are composites of men whose wives we have treated for PPD. The following story, with the exception of identifying information, is a true story about one husband's experience with two episodes of PPD. Unlike the brief cases cited here, this is one man's story from beginning to end, in his own words. We know that you will find pieces of your experience in his.

## My Wife Had Postpartum Depression: A Physician's Personal Experience

My wife has had two episodes of postpartum depression. This hardly qualifies me as an expert. I'm not a psychologist, psychiatrist, or social worker; I have no expert understanding of the workings of the human mind. I can only impart my personal experiences: what I felt, what I did, and what worked best for me.

My wife and I got married during my last year of medical school, and we decided to have our first child fairly soon after that. We had been living together for a while and felt that we were ready. For some reason, it didn't dawn on us that having a child during a medical internship might not be the wisest of ideas. Internship is, in and of itself, quite stressful—my work weeks averaged 110 to 120 hours!

Nevertheless, when our beautiful, healthy baby girl was born during the time that I had scheduled off, things seemed like they would be just fine. Initially, everything did go well. My wife was on a high, and while the baby was a little fussy, she was a joy compared to my sick patients in the hospital. After one week, I went back to work. Then the complaints began. At first, they were merely an annoyance. After all, we had a healthy baby . . . how could my wife get so upset over the baby crying a little? And so what if the baby woke up a few times in the night? "Just go back to sleep after you feed her. I do it on call in the hospital all the time," I told her. My wife would say that she couldn't fall asleep, that she couldn't do anything right.

As the complaints continued and her apparent inability to get anything done around the house deepened, I became quite confused. What should I do? Should I come home from work and take charge—hold the baby and cook dinner? When I did that, my wife complained that I made her feel inferior. Should I "play it tough" and tell my wife that she must do these things herself and refuse to help her?

The situation worsened. My wife wasn't sleeping, was constantly crying over trivial things, and was telling me that I had to stay home. "Life stayed the same for you! You get to go to work each day!" she cried.

This is where my anger kicked in. "Get to go to work?" Work, for me, meant no sleep and dying patients! Work meant being pulled in ten different directions every minute! Work meant rushing through my day to come home to being yelled at!

Unbeknownst to me, my wife was suffering from a severe case of postpartum depression. She had the insomnia and the anxiety, the feelings of helplessness, and the sense of failure. What I had was denial.

Eventually, we reached a crisis point. I could not deny the problem anymore: her doctor called me at work and told me that my wife was in need of psychiatric hospitalization—she simply couldn't function at home anymore, and outpatient treatment wasn't working. For me, the hospitalization was torture. I felt infantilized and powerless. After having learned as a doctor to expect some degree of respect in hospital settings, I was now being told whether or not I could sit on the bed with my wife or be allowed to close the door to have a private conversation. It was humiliating.

I was also attempting to balance multiple obligations. Work was and is important to me, and my fellow interns were depending on me. I wanted to be a good intern, a good father, and a good husband, but I couldn't be them all. Even though family members stepped in to help care for the baby, I still felt like I was a rubber band being stretched beyond the breaking point. I was failing as a professional, as a father, and as a husband.

I became resentful of my wife and a little jealous that she was getting all this attention and help while I was, in some perverse way, being punished for my ability to deal with the stress without totally falling apart. No one asked how I was doing. Rather, everyone seemed to make more demands of me. No matter what specific things I did to help, it wasn't enough. Somehow, I had to listen and care more. How many times can you listen to the same complaints and continue to respond with sincere and genuine compassion?

The hospitalization and subsequent recovery took several months. I was not included in the treatment plan, an exclusion that left me feeling helpless and frustrated. The care, however, was progressive in other ways. For example, my wife was allowed daily visits with the baby, making a normal mother-baby relationship possible. Over time, my wife returned to her old self, and so did I. Soon, with PPD past us, life's other more immediately pressing problems commanded my attention. Amidst residency and raising a child, I didn't take time to think about PPD anymore.

My reactions to the first episode have several main features. First of all, despite my medical training, I was totally ignorant of postpartum depression. I had no idea what was happening and hadn't been prepared to expect that it would happen. Second, there was a tremendous amount of job stress creating conflicting obligations. Last, I had virtually no emotional support. This is scarcely surprising—I believe that I am like many other men, in that I have only one best friend whom I trust with my deepest fears and insecurities—my wife. She wasn't there; this illness was. Moreover, this wasn't something I was likely to confide in other, lesser friends, because of the stigma that is attached to mental illnesses in our society. For that same reason, my family was not as supportive as they would have been if my wife had suffered, say, an automobile accident. My wife's psychiatrist was concerned about her. His job was not to monitor my welfare. But even if "help" had been offered, it would have been impossible for me to accept, because lack of time was my greatest stressor.

Three-and-a-half years later, we had a second child. By now my wife and I had both become quite informed regarding PPD. We knew what it was and what it was not. Although we knew that there was a risk of recurrence, we thought that we would sail through having another baby. "Things are different now," we thought. My wife was an experienced mother and comfortable in her role. She had a network of supportive friends who were parents and who were knowledgeable about PPD. I'd be around much more.

When our second daughter was born, it seemed that we had been right. The situation was ideal; the baby was perfect. She slept through the night from day one and beamed whenever my wife was near. She hardly ever cried. In my opinion, what happened next was exclusively biological. All at once, it seemed like a switch flipped in my wife's brain. One night—suddenly—she couldn't sleep. The same the next night, and then the terrible anxiety kicked in.

Medication was administered early, but it still was three months until the depression resolved significantly. One medication had side effects and needed to be stopped. Another just plain didn't work after the trial period.

Having our older daughter around was a mixed blessing. It was more complicated to get substitute caretakers to cover for two children, but she also helped to enforce a routine on the household. She provided a very valuable distraction.

I cannot speak to how the second episode felt for my wife, but to me, the experiences were like night and day. This time we were not ignorant about PPD. I was not annoyed or confused; I was concerned and hopeful that recovery would occur quickly. I only experienced significant frustration when my wife didn't recover as quickly as I thought she was supposed to. Yes, I was angry that it happened again, but not angry at her. This time I knew it wasn't her fault.

I was not totally powerless this time, either. There were things I could do that I knew were appreciated. While the things I did could not make it all better, they did make a difference. I still had conflicting obligations at work, but much less so than with the first episode. There was some emotional support for me this time; people asked me how I was doing. Also, my wife's knowledge of PPD allowed her to keep some objectivity and not be swallowed up by this illness; I could still talk to her.

Unfortunately, I think that few fathers know about PPD, about how common it is and what to expect as it runs its course. Without this information, we have no idea about what we can or should do and often may fear that our wives will never be better. We may be shocked to learn that at least 10 percent of mothers experience a severe form of PPD and that they do get better again. We have to confront our own prejudices against mental illnesses, then deal with the preconceptions that others have about mental illness and about motherhood. And then there's the unsolicited advice: "It's all in her head," "She's just being lazy," "Tell her to stop whining and just do it," "It's because you do too much for her." People don't understand mental illness and, as always, are afraid of what they do not understand.

We fathers also feel a tremendous sense of powerlessness. These events are mostly out of our control. No matter what we do, our wives are still depressed and anxious. This feeling is exacerbated, because we are typically being excluded from the treatment plan. Decisions are made without our input or knowledge, and often we are left adrift without any guidance. We want to do something to help, but almost anything we do seems to make things worse. For many, the financial stress of paying for therapy, medication, and hospitalization makes you feel all the more helpless.

Most of us work hard to get where we are in our jobs and pride ourselves on feeling that our coworkers can depend on us. In many workplaces, there is very little "give" for family crises. The demands of having a wife with PPD may threaten our very ability to provide for our family. And there usually isn't anyone you can talk to about the pressures. While there are built-in supports around other family crises—the rituals that accompany mourning guarantee that we'll have people to lean on, for example—with this crisis, a father suffers alone and in silence, afraid even to tell his wife how much it hurts him to see her suffering so.

But we don't need to be ignorant, helpless creatures. The most important tool we have is knowledge. We must educate both ourselves and those who are important to us about PPD. They must learn that PPD is not a woman being lazy or crazy and that, despite sensationalistic talk shows implying otherwise, having PPD does not mean that she is going to kill the baby or herself. It is a treatable medical illness, like diabetes, and she will get better.

You can help your wife. Reassure her, again and again and again. "You will get better." "You will get through it." She will.

You can also help by doing what needs to be done around the house and for the baby. Ask her what specific things she wants you to do. Just as importantly, provide only the level of support she requests, so that she can do those things that she wants to do for herself. Achieving this balance can be difficult. You may find yourself measuring and setting out the ingredients so that she is able to cook dinner. Or getting the bath and clothes set up so that she can bathe and dress the baby. Ask for guidance from her and her therapist.

Remember though: you cannot make her better; only time and proper treatment will do that. The disease is not your fault or her fault. You can help yourself by knowing your own limits and finding someone to cover for you, so you can get out once in a while. Perhaps one of her friends can come over for an evening, or a family member can help out. You can't take care of her if you fall apart yourself.

PPD is absolutely awful for mothers, but it is hard on fathers, too. There may be no one to support you but yourself. Don't forget to do it. PPD may last weeks or months. But when it's over, you have your wife and child for your lifetime.

# 11

# "THIS IS SUPPOSED TO BE THE BEST TIME IN MY LIFE"

## *Fantasies and Expectations of Motherhood*

*. . . But tell me,*
*I'm not the only one am I?*
*There must be others like me who*
*in the early hours*
*empty their breasts and swear*
*this is the last,*
*not another drop more . . .*

—JANE SCHAPIRO, "POSTPARTUM"

ALL WOMEN APPROACH the transition to motherhood with preconceived ideas based on their own life experiences and cultural background. Expectations and fantasies are a natural and healthy way of preparing for motherhood. When you fantasize about something, you actually form a mental image of how you expect it to be. The technique of forming this mental image or "walking" yourself through the imagined steps of an unknown process is a very successful strategy for coping with and preparing for any new experience. By storing subconscious thoughts and images in this way, you have been preparing for motherhood for some time.

But when there is a significant discrepancy between what you anticipate and what you actually experience, guilt, confusion, and great unhappiness can result. No mother comes out of childbirth unchanged; even the happiest of new mothers has some disappointments. When you have PPD, a more acute trauma is caused by the increased quantity and severity of those disappointments—no woman with PPD experiences the initial stages of motherhood as she had fantasized. Making matters worse, your weakened psychological state prevents you from dealing with those disappointments in your usual way. Unfulfilled expectations, unanticipated losses, and lack of support create a potential for PPD to develop if a woman is biochemically predisposed. Once PPD has taken hold, a woman will feel these pains more intensely, especially as she develops the exaggerated tendency toward self-criticism and heightened emotional sensitivity that are symptomatic of depression.

The following three chapters address issues related to some of the expectations and visions of motherhood that characterize this transition. When you are recovering from PPD, you must come to terms with your unfulfilled expectations and fantasies, understand the disappointments and losses that you feel, and adapt to a new self-image and identity. As the process of recovery from PPD continues, it may entail the reconciliation of issues raised between yourself and your own parents. Exploration of these issues should only be tackled after you have mobilized your resources for support and begun to feel some relief.

This next step in the recovery process is one of introspection and self-examination. One of the most effective methods to help women with PPD gain understanding about why they feel the way they do about motherhood is to recall and analyze some of the mental images that have been collected over an entire lifetime.

## Cultural Expectations of Motherhood

Sarah, who is four months pregnant, hopes she'll be a perfect mother, "When I have this baby, I'm going to say all the right things, make all the right choices, and help make this world a wonderful and safe place for my baby to live." If you believe what you see in television commercials and magazine advertisements, every mother has a perfectly flawless infant with a twinkle in his eyes and a smile of contentment on his face. His mother wakes happily to feed him. She is always rested, and her makeup is always in place. She places the baby to her breast as they both gaze meaningfully into each others' eyes. They bond instantly.

But by now, you have discovered the reality behind the Gerber Baby myth—the incessant crying, the endless dirty diapers, the sleepless nights. Society reinforces the myth of the perfect baby in the arms of the perfect mother, with all her maternal instincts intact. In previous years, there was so much emphasis on the phenomenon of "bonding" that women often plummeted into despair when they failed to feel an instant love attachment to this blessed creature. As one mother stated: "I wept as I looked into those sweet blue eyes. Who is this little person? Do I know you?"

Our culture and the media play a powerful role in shaping our expectations. And these expectations, in turn, create enormous pressure on mothers to strive for perfection. Think about some of the television shows that center on family life. Many overglamorize motherhood, placing it high on a pedestal for all to admire, or reinforce the illusion that we can all strive for supermom status. Others actually demean a mother's role by setting us up to laugh at how overwhelmed, disorganized, or disoriented she is in a variety of "real-life" situations. When producers of television programming or movies respond to the criticism that these "Hollywood" depictions of mothers do not represent realistic portrayals, they typically justify their position by claiming that if it were realistic, it wouldn't be 100 percent entertaining. How true!

## Childhood Expectations of Motherhood

Our images of ourselves as mothers begin very early in our psychological development. By the age of two or three, little girls start to identify with their mothers and see themselves as potential mothers. The expectation of becoming mothers when we grew up permeated our childhood play—before we even knew where babies came from, most of us were dressing up as Mommy and playing "house"—and shaped our sense of what being female would mean to us.

Take a moment and go way back in time. Picture yourself playing with dolls. What did the mommy doll do? What did she say? Was she happy? What was the baby doll like? Did it cry? Did it sleep? Was it perfect?

If these memories are hard to reach, watch a young girl play now. As mothers of daughters, we can tell you that things haven't changed so much. Though we may try to expose our daughters to toys with little or no specific gender orientation, our daughters wear the fanciest pretend clothes, never forget lipstick or nail polish, and have perfectly coordinated and compliant baby dolls who gaze lovingly at their "Mommies" while peacefully resting in their "cribs." How many times have you heard a young girl say that when she grows up, she wants to be a mommy, sometimes, "more than anything else in the whole wide world."

Since many of the most fundamental images we have about motherhood have been with us since childhood and are deeply ingrained, we can't help but idealize motherhood when we become adults and mothers ourselves. Often, our later experiences only seem to consolidate these infantile idealizations. For example, when we babysat as teenagers, most of us began with older (easier) babies, and never so much as glimpsed the difficulties of dealing with an infant.

## Adult Expectations of Motherhood

Many women remember attaching some specific expectation to their decision to have a baby. Earlier in this chapter we introduced Sarah, who had visions of being the perfect mother. She often repeated her strong conviction that she would be the "kind of mother I never had." Sarah secretly hoped that this baby would help bring her closer to her mother, with whom she had a strained relationship. Once she discovered the magic potion for becoming the perfect mother, she would be able to fill in the gaps left from her own upbringing.

Many women, like Sarah, silently hope that having a baby will consolidate a weak relationship or bring harmony to their lives in some way. Consider the women who think that having a baby will bring them closer to their husbands. Or did you perhaps believe that having a baby would make your family or your husband's family happy, especially if you had a boy who could carry on the family name? Some women feel that having a baby provides an entree into private adult circles and that becoming a parent carries with it a certain social status that is shared only by other couples with children. These and other prenatal fantasies directly impact how you feel after the baby is born. Unconsciously, we try to match our actual experience with our previous expectation, and as we have already noted, the discrepancy between them creates tension and internal conflict.

One of the best ways to access your original baby fantasy and assess its associated expectation/loss component is to recall what you thought when you first learned you were pregnant. It is important to note that if your pregnancy was long-awaited or difficult to achieve, your expectations may have been especially great and perhaps attained particular psychological importance.

Do you remember how you felt when you discovered you were pregnant? Excited? Nervous? Happy? Scared? You probably felt a little bit of everything. If you remember one feeling as being more prominent than the others, try to focus on that feeling for a moment. What was the first thing you thought after you felt so nervous or so excited? What did you do? Who was the first person you told? Do you remember what it was like when you told your husband, your parents, your best friend? Sarah remembered calling her friend after they'd both found out they were pregnant around the same time. They laughed as they fantasized about strolling through the park on spring days, breastfeeding their babies in all kinds of public places, fixing their children up for dates if one had a boy and one had a girl. Everything was going to be perfectly wonderful.

## When Expectations Are Not Met: Ambivalence and Disappointment

The fantasies we have about the kind of mother we will be have a tremendous impact on how we feel once we become mothers, as they set us up to believe that we have to behave and respond and feel a certain way. When our reactions do not live up to these ideals, we feel as though we have failed.

This sense of failure is based on a polarized, black-or-white, right-or-wrong perspective. But real life has shades of gray. One of the first steps you need to take to overcome your self-defeating disappointment is to accept your ambivalence. Ambivalence is defined as the existence of mutually conflicting emotions. It means you can love your baby, yet also feel let down. It means you can enjoy being a mother while simultaneously missing your friends at work and wondering why you are home instead.

Although it is natural to have contradictory feelings imposed on us by motherhood, it is just as natural for a woman to be frustrated by these feelings. To acknowledge ambivalence is not an expression of failure. Nor does it challenge the investment we all have in being the best mother we can. It simply means we can feel good and bad at once. We can love our baby and feel angry at the same time. We can love being a mother and resent giving up our free time. Though we are taught to search for and embrace the positive feelings that prevail, every mother, whether or not she has PPD, has experienced these ambivalent feelings at one time or another.

## Our Romanticized Self as Mother

Once you understand why expectations carry so much emotional weight, you can appreciate why one of the major steps to recovery is healing from your own unrealized fantasies. Try to be as specific as possible when you answer the following questions. You might find it more comfortable to think in terms of a "third person" context, referring to "she" and "her," instead of "I" and "my." This will also help to provide you with more objectivity. Let your imagination carry you back to your memory of that perfect mother you wanted so very much to be. What would she be like? How would she act? What would she look like? Try to create a detailed image: she will always have a clean house; she will always put her baby's needs before her own; she will always dress casually, but be neat and pressed; she will continue to have romantic and sexual adventures with her husband; she will love to sit for hours and play one-on-one with her baby.

My Romanticized Self as Mother

1. _____
2. _____
3. _____
4. _____
5. _____
6. _____
7. _____
8. _____

Now make a list based on the "real" mother you see yourself as every day. Try not to be too hard on yourself and remain as objective as possible. Be sure to do this part of the exercise with a "first person" pronoun so you can relate better: sometimes my house is cluttered, and I have often gone a week without doing any laundry; I usually wear old sweat clothes around the house; my husband and I haven't made love in a while, but we are trying to touch and say nice things to each other as often as possible; when I don't feel like playing with my baby, I put her in her playpen so she can play alone while I do something else.

The Reality of Myself as Mother

1. _____
2. _____
3. _____
4. _____
5. _____
6. _____
7. _____
8. _____

Go back and compare the two lists. What does this teach us? Remember, it is the discrepancy between them that is causing some of your pain. The following pages illustrate specific areas in which discrepancies between fantasy and reality frequently occur. Later in this chapter, we will address the process of learning how to minimize these discrepancies in order to reduce the inner conflict and pain.

## Romanticization of Childbirth and Early Motherhood

Fantasies about pregnancy and motherhood often include dreams, wishes, and hopes about different aspects of the childbirth experience. Start by thinking about the fantasies you had about what labor and delivery would be like. Then reflect on your actual experience. Most likely, there will be some discrepancy between these two recollections that can contribute to an overall positive or negative emotional state. Some women have found childbirth to be an exhilarating process that surpassed their wildest imaginings. Other women feel disappointed, ashamed, deprived, angry, or sad about their experience of labor and delivery.

If you had a negative childbirth experience, be assured—you are not alone. The following statements are by other women who were disappointed, too:

- I thought that since I would have an epidural, it wouldn't hurt. I didn't know that they wouldn't put it in until I was almost done with labor. It was excruciating.
- I pictured a totally natural delivery in the birthing center. I can't believe I ended up with induced labor, a caesarian section, a huge scar, and a baby who had to be resuscitated. It makes me feel like there's something wrong with my body, because I couldn't give birth naturally.
- I'm embarrassed about how I lost control. I felt like a sweaty, filthy, primitive animal. My husband teases me, but I don't have any sense of humor about it at all. It was the worst experience of my life.

Other women are let down by their fantasies about what the first few minutes with their baby would be like:

- I was so looking forward to breastfeeding—I'd heard about how nursing on the delivery table helped your uterus go back down. Forget it—my baby never really nursed right for a week. Instead of this blissful experience, every time I put him to my breast we both cried hysterically. I was at the pediatrician's for weight checks every day for a week! I'm not sure I'd go through that again.

* I pictured this great moment of bonding with my infant. We'd gaze into each other's eyes, and the love would flow. I just didn't feel it—I have to admit that it took a while to feel anything toward that funny-looking creature.

Other women are disappointed by their fantasies about what the first few weeks of sharing parenthood with their husband would be like:

* We had always had a modern type of marriage when it came to housework. Suddenly, he went into this macho hunter-gatherer mode, working constantly and talking about how much money he needed to save for our baby daughter's wedding. I feel like our marriage went back in time twenty-five years.

## Other Disappointments

### PREVIOUS PREGNANCY-RELATED LOSS

If you have experienced a previous miscarriage, stillbirth, or abortion, or if you have had infertility problems or a family history of pregnancy-related loss, it is important to understand how much impact these experiences can have on your decision to get pregnant and your experience of pregnancy and childbirth. What may not be so easy to understand is that these factors may also affect the way you feel after your baby is born. Although it seems that the birth of a baby after a previous loss could only be received as a welcome and blessed event, often it is complicated by the emergence of unresolved anger, guilt, or sadness over the previous loss.

Women with PPD who have suffered a previous pregnancy-related loss tell us they feel a disproportionate amount of grief after the birth of their baby. A woman once described her aunt's reaction to the birth of her son after several miscarriages: "After so much sadness, you have been blessed with such a beautiful baby. It is unthinkable that you are not appreciating every moment you have with your loved one." It is not easy for you or for others to understand why you may be feeling so let down at a time when you "should" be feeling such pleasure. The birth of your baby can actually generate feelings of grief over the previous loss(es), creating a state of discontent and confusion. When you are depressed, normal grief reactions are exaggerated and difficult to put in perspective. We suggest consulting a therapist to help you sort out these complex emotions, as your awareness and confrontation of these unresolved feelings can help relieve this pain over time.

## IF YOUR PREGNANCY WASN'T PLANNED

One of the hardest issues to work through after childbirth is facing ambivalence about what was once an unwanted or unplanned pregnancy. As one mother said, "How can I love my baby so much right now when a year ago I was considering an abortion?" Others who may not have considered abortion will remember the terrible sinking feeling they had when the pregnancy was confirmed. This same feeling may reemerge after childbirth as part of the guilt so common in PPD. In other words, since having PPD predisposes you to excessive feelings of guilt, you are likely to be quite hard on yourself if the pregnancy was unplanned. "Maybe I'm feeling so depressed because I didn't want to have another baby, and now I'm being punished." Try to keep in mind: when your pregnancy was discovered, you reacted to an idea— the idea of being pregnant and having a baby. You did not react to this person who is now in your family. Nature allows pregnant women nine months to readjust and anticipate this change. You did not cause your PPD by wishing at one point that you were not pregnant.

## SPECIAL CIRCUMSTANCES

There are a number of other circumstances that can make a mother susceptible to a period of emotional upheaval after the birth of her child, including giving birth to a premature or handicapped baby and having an emergency caesarian section.

Obstetric and pediatric complications do increase vulnerability to PPD. Women who have birth-related traumas are certainly going to experience postpartum stress. Unfortunately, they often go through much of it alone. Whenever something bad happens to a baby—everyone seems to disappear. People don't know how to respond. They are often afraid they will say the wrong thing, so they often don't say or do anything.

These mothers are at risk for serious emotional strain, and although they are understandably preoccupied with the well-being of their baby, many of them need to be gently reminded to take care of themselves. One important way is to take advantage of self-help and support organizations that are available.

## Letting Go of Your Expectations

In treatment, Ellen talks about the expectations she had about how her baby would affect her marriage:

> I can't believe it, but I really thought having this baby would make such a difference to Paul. I thought that the strain in our marriage would somehow miraculously fade, and we would fall into a nice, peaceful rhythm. But nothing has changed. It was hard for me to accept this, but now I'm sure that the problems we had before are still very much here. When I'm not feeling so incredibly angry, I feel lonely. Where is my perfect marriage?

Women with PPD have a more difficult time letting go of unfulfilled expectations, because their resources are weakened and perceptions may be distorted. Previously we saw how easy it is to get stuck in negative modes of thinking. Sometimes, you can get so caught up in the cycle of despair that you can no longer distinguish objective reality from your own pessimistic distortion. For instance, while a mother who is up three-quarters of the night with a sick infant may still think she should feel alert and relaxed the next day, it is obvious to onlookers that this is not a realistic expectation for anyone. But because she is already feeling so inadequate and unsure of herself, she resists admitting her exhaustion and need for help.

In order to reframe your expectations successfully, you must first break down the original expectations into components. The following exercise and example will walk you through the process of reframing the expectations that may be creating pressure for you.

Step 1. **Identify the expectation:** *"I had hoped my baby would be quiet and easy to care for."*

Step 2. **Acknowledge the reality:** *"My baby is fussy and hard to soothe."*

Step 3. **Identify your feeling:** *"This makes me frustrated and tense."*

Step 4. **Support and accept your feeling:** *"No wonder I'm so upset. It's hard to take care of a fussy baby!"*

Step 5. **State your loss:** *"I don't have a quiet, easy baby."*

Step 6. **Refocus statement:** *"My baby is spirited and is very independent."*

As you read through this above illustration, think about how you might feel if this example pertained to you. When you "acknowledge the reality" in Step 2, do you feel agitated? When you "identify your feeling" in Step 3, do you feel a sense of self-righteousness? When you "support and accept your feeling" in Step 4, can you feel a hint of relief? When you "state your loss" in Step 5, do you feel disappointed or sad? And when you "refocus the statement" in Step 6, do you feel a sense of resignation, or maybe even pride?

Here is another example:

I expected that having a baby would affect my relationship with my husband by . . .

Step 1.  *I thought that my husband and I would get very close after we had the baby.*

Step 2.  *My husband has to work hard and come home late in the evening.*

Step 3.  *I miss time alone with my husband. I am angry and lonely.*

Step 4.  *It's no wonder I feel so angry and lonely after being with the baby all day long. Anyone would feel this way day after day.*

Step 5.  *My husband and I have less time together than ever before.*

Step 6.  *My husband and I will have to make a special effort to find time alone without the baby, so we can feel good about each other again.*

Now try this exercise using the above example of an expectation about your husband that was not met, or use the following: I expected that being a mother would feel . . .

Successfully letting go of your fantasies and expectations does not mean you're going to like the way it feels at first, and it does not mean you won't feel sad about giving up those expectations. What you are doing here is making room for alternative reasoning and emotions. As we saw in Chapter 3, when you have PPD, it is very easy to slip into negative thought patterns. Interrupting this cycle is one of the most effective ways for you to take control over how you are feeling. When you are used to thinking and feeling a certain way, it will initially feel awkward to "force" yourself to think and feel differently. But you'll be amazed how well it works! As one woman put it, "It's like I'm doing everything with my left hand instead of my right. I know it will work, it just feels a little funny."

## Your Drive to Be the Perfect Mother

When you expect perfection, you are setting yourself up for failure. Many women who remember periods of chaos or unmet needs from their childhoods promise themselves that they will do everything to prevent that pattern from repeating itself with their own child. The very primary desire to have a perfect mother now compels you to be a perfect mother. And so you set out to meet the needs that were left unmet by your own mother to fill the gaps, to right the wrongs.

The danger here is that this goal cannot possibly be attained, so you will inevitably perceive your performance as a failure. You must make room for adaptations, modifications, experimentation, and—perhaps most important—mistakes. In the long run, these shortcomings won't seem so earth-shattering. Human beings are very resilient, and despite overblown pseudo-psychology, letting your baby sit in a wet diaper for a half hour or forgetting to sterilize a nipple is not going to scar him for life. If you have significant unresolved needs from your childhood, please consider therapy. Expecting to repair the past by becoming a perfect mother is a sure way to set yourself up for disappointment.

Remember that women learn to become good mothers by trial and error, by struggling through the daily demands of caring for their babies, by doing some things right, and by making some mistakes.

## Give Yourself Some Credit

Women with PPD tend to be very hard on themselves, so it is especially important for you to give yourself permission to make mistakes. Making a list of the things you think you are doing wrong would be easy. Instead, why don't you try to make a list of some of the things you are doing right that you haven't given yourself credit for. In other words, in what ways are you a good mother and in what ways are you living up to your expectations for yourself? Don't forget to give yourself credit for small achievements:

*Examples:* My baby is always clean.

I take my baby for walks in the stroller.

1. _____

2. _____

3. _____

4. _____
5. _____

If you can't think of anything to write down, try to pinpoint some of the tasks you are doing by instinct, and you are not giving yourself credit for. You must give yourself credit for every little thing you are doing.

- What about feeding the baby? How do you know what and how much to feed? Is he gaining weight?
- What do you do to try to soothe your baby? Does it work? How do you know?
- Do you know when your baby is hungry? How does he signal you?
- Do you ever hold your baby just to feel close to him, even when he isn't crying?
- How does your baby like to fall asleep? What is his favorite position? If someone else was trying to get your baby to sleep, what would they need to know?

These are just a few examples of some of the ways you are being a successful mother that you may have just picked up along the way. Just think, you didn't know any of this before!

Remember, there is no script for this performance, no instruction manual, and there are very few guidelines. You are probably your harshest critic. Be kind to yourself and remember that you are doing the best you can. Try not to compare yourself to other mothers, your mother, or the perfect mothers you see on TV!

## Focus on Positive Feelings

Now that you've identified some real practical success, think about the positive side of your emotional state. Does anything feel good

about being a new mother? If you can find some good feelings related to any part of your new role as mother, write them down. It is
human nature to worry about the ways in which we are feeling unfulfilled or disappointed. But sometimes, we forget to take notice of
the simple ways that we feel good. It is important not to lose sight of
these, no matter how unrelated or insignificant you may think they
are. Remember that women without PPD have more fun and enjoy-
able experiences to counterbalance the disappointment than women
with PPD.

What feels good to you right now? Anything? Here are some
examples:

- I like holding my baby and resting with him first thing in
  the morning.
- I like being able to understand what my baby needs at cer-
  tain times.
- I love having a "family."
- I love to call my old friends and trade stories about our
  babies.
- I love to stare at my baby while he sleeps in his crib.

1. _____
2. _____
3. _____
4. _____
5. _____

Refer to this list when you need to. Change it. Add to it. Cross
things out—whatever you have to do to keep it current. Keeping track
of the intermittent good feelings that may sneak in actually helps you
to integrate them and break negative thought cycles.

Letting go and reframing your expectations is not easy. Try not to
be discouraged if it feels beyond your grasp. Like any new experience,

after some initial resistance and accommodations, you will find it gets more natural in time. Don't worry about the length of time it takes for you to feel comfortable with these exercises. Mastering these skills could take days, weeks, or months. Every time you practice one of them, you are incorporating a new skill that will help you in the long run as well as today.

# 12

# "What Happened to That Person I Used to Be?"

*Exploring Your Losses and Reclaiming Your Self-Esteem*

> *As for our losses and gains, we have seen how often they are inextricably mixed. There is plenty we have to give up in order to grow. For we cannot deeply love anything without becoming vulnerable to loss.*
>
> —Judith Viorst, *Necessary Losses*

*W*HEN PEOPLE THINK ABOUT having babies, they usually think in terms of what will be gained: a new baby who will carry on the family name and family traditions, a source of joy and pride, the embodiment of ones hopes and dreams.

But along with the gains come some very real losses. Our culture doesn't readily acknowledge these losses, but all mothers experience them to some extent, and when they do, they often feel cheated and isolated. Even though these feelings are universal, women with PPD will find adapting to these losses especially difficult because of their increased physical and emotional vulnerability.

It is not easy to reconcile the sadness and vulnerability that accompany the birth of a child. To some extent, we all have a mental picture of the idealized version of maternal love, characterized by total selflessness and abandonment of personal needs and interests. It is safe, nonjudgmental, ever present, and ever powerful. We all yearned for this type of maternal love when we were children, and we want to provide it now for our children. Having to give up this romanticized image of the perfect mother-baby relationship is one of the losses that come with the early stages of mothering.

Many women with PPD tell us that they just don't feel like themselves. Part of what they are saying is that their image of themselves is changing. They are responding to their surroundings in new ways, with new feelings that can be very forceful and unsettling. One of our goals in this chapter is to help you rediscover parts of your self-identity that seem to be temporarily out of reach. This process has several steps. The first is to acknowledge your losses: to understand that no matter what anyone tries to tell you, you have definitely experienced some monumental losses that need to be addressed. After you have taken a closer look at some of the things you have given up, you will learn how necessary it is to mourn some of these losses by identifying the feelings associated with them. You will also learn how important it is to accept the presence of these negative feelings in order to make room for new positive ones, and to lay the groundwork for you to begin to like yourself again. Finally, after some discussion on coming to terms with these losses, we will explore the concept of self-esteem and how to revitalize yourself.

## Acknowledging Your Losses

Acknowledging the losses you have experienced is important for several reasons. This process of understanding what you have given up will validate some of the pain you feel. It will reassure you that these feelings are not unusual, and it will minimize the guilt that may be compounding the pain.

A mother of a new baby may lose:

- Spontaneity
- Self-confidence
- Independence
- Control
- Predictability
- Security
- Money
- Sleep
- Her physical shape
- Self-identity
- Couple time
- Her career
- Time for herself
- Intimacy
- The dream of being a perfect mother
- Sexuality
- The special attention of being pregnant
- The dream of having a perfect baby
- Adult company

This partial list may include many of the things that help make you feel good about yourself. Admitting these losses does not in any way mean that you do not appreciate how special your new baby is or that you are not a wonderful mother. Instead, admitting them represents a shift in the equilibrium of your life events. When we experience something new, different, and challenging, we have to make room for it in our life. Often, this accommodation is made by giving something else up, even temporarily.

The sudden changes brought on by becoming a mother are illustrated in the case of Ellen, a nurse who was three months postpartum when she described what she called "the devastation of motherhood":

> I was so used to feeling in charge of my life. Things made sense and were somewhat predictable. Everything had its place. Then, I had a baby. Suddenly, I find myself in this new place, with spit-up all over me. I haven't washed my hair in four days, because I haven't had five minutes to take a shower. I've been eating fast food for weeks, and I don't have the nerve to ask my husband to do a load of laundry. I haven't left the house in days, and I can't even remember when I got more than two hours of sleep in a row. And I wonder why I feel so out of control?

Ellen's testimony demonstrates how rapidly things can fall apart. Many losses—control, predictability, time for self, sleep, independence, physical shape, and so on—will combine to create a picture of frenzy and confusion. Each loss represents an area of your life that held special meaning to you, and when you experience several losses at a time, you can be quickly and quite understandably overwhelmed.

Take a look at a few of the losses from the list more closely, and as you read the questions in each of the following sections, be aware of how many you would answer "yes" to. Each one you respond affirmatively to represents another way you have lost a little more, and it will become clear that their impact on your self-identity has been very real. As you think about the sacrifices that have become so much a part of your life, it will make sense that you will sometimes feel sad during a time when society, your friends, your family, and most of all you, expect you to feel happy. These are examples of how much you have given up:

Independence:

- Remember when you and your husband could pick up and go out to dinner just because you felt like it?

❀ Remember when you could run back to the grocery store because you forgot one item, without having to deal with the snowsuit, mittens, hat, car seat, and bottle?

Sleep:
❀ Before the baby, did you sleep for seven or eight uninterrupted hours?
❀ Did you enjoy sleeping late on weekends?

Physical Shape:
❀ Did you like the way you looked before you got pregnant?
❀ Do you wish you could look like that again now?
❀ Are you amazed at how quickly other mothers seem to regain their pre-pregnant shape?

Self-Identity:
❀ Do you ever catch yourself saying, "I never used to do this the way I do now," or "I always used to do that but now I can't"?
❀ Are people close to you making comments about how different you seem, look, or act?
❀ Do you find yourself making excuses or compromising more than you would like to?

Career:
❀ Were you working for five, ten, fifteen, or twenty years before you decided to have a baby?
❀ If you plan to return to your job, how much time are you taking off?
❀ If you've already returned to work in any capacity, do you feel pulled in several directions? Are you constantly reorganizing your priorities? Do you feel guilty about being at

work when you're there? Do you feel guilty about not working hard enough when you're not there?

- If you haven't returned to work, do you feel like you
  have "baby brains" and miss the stimulation of adult
  interactions?

Time for Self:

(Most women say, "Time for myself? What's that?")

- Do you constantly feel like you are running and doing for
  everyone else?
- Do you ever do nice things just for yourself?
- Do you feel selfish or guilty if you admit that there is something you want or need?

Dream of Being a Perfect Mother:

- Did you have any unexpected complications during your
  pregnancy or delivery?
- Did you discover rather abruptly that things just weren't
  going to go the way you thought they would?
- Were you surprised to learn that your baby would not be
  perfect, that he would cry out incessantly for your immediate attention when you had nothing left to give?
- Have you felt tired, cranky, insecure, or misunderstood
  since the birth of your baby?
- Are you forever reflecting about how you hoped it would
  be?

Dream of Having a Perfect Baby:

- Have you heard all those stories about women who started
  businesses from their homes while their two-month-olds
  slept peacefully nearby?
- And what about the tales of little ones who play for hours
  in the playpen while Mommy and Daddy entertain guests?

## Taking Inventory of Your Losses

When you recognize what you have lost, you will begin to understand some of your sadness and will have taken the first step toward overcoming it. Remember: *acknowledging the losses that come with a new baby does not mean that you don't love your baby*.

What do you miss the most? What losses are most significant to you? Refer to the previous list or use your own:

1. _____
2. _____
3. _____
4. _____
5. _____

Acknowledging these losses may be very difficult for you. Giving up parts of yourself that were comfortable and gave you a sense of self-worth is naturally hard to do. To make matters worse, everything seems to be lost at once, magnifying the pain.

Look over your list and honestly ask yourself whether these losses are permanent or irrevocable. Put a check mark next to any loss that is absolutely gone forever. (We predict that you won't have more than one.) For the most part, these losses are temporary. Although it feels like your time, flexibility, sexual energy, whatever, are gone for good, don't worry, they'll be back.

## Grieving Your Losses

"I've changed so much. I was looking through my photo album last night and ran across pictures of my honeymoon. I looked so pretty, so skinny, so happy. I miss who I used to be. I don't feel like myself anymore."

Much of the sorrow you feel during this period of transition is a reaction to your changing self. When you have PPD, these changes are particularly disturbing, as now is a time when you crave consistency and predictability. It feels like part of yourself is lost forever. Cindy, the mother of a fourteen-month-old, recollects how she felt about herself.

"I used to be so laid back, nothing ever bothered me. Then before I knew it, every little thing started to get on my nerves. I became so irritable and miserable to live with, I was afraid my husband would get tired of coming home. I didn't think I would ever feel like my old self again."

It may help you deal with your confusion and unhappiness to understand that part of the process you must go through to recover from postpartum losses is similar to the mourning process when someone dies. When someone dies, one stage of grieving is characterized by focusing on the lost person. We get out old photographs, talk about who this person was, reminisce and tell stories that start with "Remember when . . ." It's as if in order to absorb the loss, we need to review each painful memory. Although it hurts, this process can also offer consolation and comfort to ease the loss. Similarly, when you have PPD, you, too, will be comforted by the bittersweet memories of your not-so-distant past.

Take a minute and think about the "old you" that you miss so much. What was she like? Can you describe her on a typical day? It may help to get out some photographs to tell yourself her story. What did she look like? How would you describe her personality? How did she feel? What did she do? What do you miss most about her?

As you think about this former image of yourself, try to be aware of how it makes you feel. Does it make you sad when you think of how you used to be? Does it make you feel angry or scared? Confronting these feelings is an important step in the grief process, as you mourn for parts of your previous self.

Go back to the list of losses that you identified earlier and try to recognize how each loss makes you feel. Be as specific as possible:

| Loss | Makes Me Feel |
|------|---------------|
| Example: *Friends at work* | *lonely* |
| 1. _____ | _____ |
| 2. _____ | _____ |
| 3. _____ | _____ |
| 4. _____ | _____ |
| 5. _____ | _____ |

What do you do with these feelings? Most likely, you have tried to tuck them away, because you couldn't bear to admit you felt them. It is frightening to picture yourself resenting your baby, getting mad at your husband, or thinking that it was a terrible mistake to have the baby at this time. But be assured, most mothers do feel angry at their babies and angry at their partners, at times.

As we discussed in Chapter 3, you must permit yourself to have negative feelings. If you do not admit you are experiencing some negative feelings as a result of these losses, you are likely to develop a defense reaction that may get in the way of your effort to deal with your emotions. In an effort to protect yourself from feeling the emotional vulnerability and pain, you may end up worsening your PPD by directing the anger, resentment, and sadness back toward yourself. Denying negative feelings also keeps you from exploring ways to compensate for the losses that caused them.

The sadness you might feel right now is a healthy and natural part of the grieving process we referred to that you must go through in order to recover from these losses. This part of the recovery process is always difficult for women to understand. We often hear women say, "Why do I have to make myself feel so bad in order to feel better? Wasn't I better off before I started thinking about all these things that make me so sad all the time?" These questions actually refer to a core principle of therapy that we talked about in earlier chapters: it takes much more energy to stuff negative feelings inside than it does to confront them. Only after you have brought negative feelings to light can you safely put them away in a place that will no longer impede your recovery.

## Coming to Terms with a Loss

Sometimes the losses we feel are so private and personal that it is difficult to believe that someone else could possibly understand what we are feeling. While writing this book, Karen recalled what she felt when her son was born:

There was no doubt in my mind that I would have a beautiful baby. I remember picturing him in my head while I was pregnant: a cross between my brother, my sister, and myself. It was as if I knew what he would look like even before he was born.

But after being three weeks post due and having his head engaged in my pelvis for that extended period of time, my baby was born, via caesarian, with a pronounced "cone head." His skull had been squeezed for too long, his Apgar score was 2, and they whisked him away from me. After being reassured that he was fine, I remember holding him for the first time in the recovery room. I looked at his crying eyes and his sweet face. And his head. It was horrible. All the doctors told me it was normal and that it would regain its proper shape in a couple of weeks. It did not—it would take a year.

I asked the nurses to bring me a little cap for his head. I gently covered his misshapen head and kept that cap on his head for days while I nursed him. He looked perfect that way.

Up until the moment my son was born, I carried my dream of having a perfect baby. That dream was superseded by the loss I felt during the early days after his birth. I learned quickly that the loss can coexist with the unconditional love I felt for him, and I was able to give myself completely to my child. No one likes admitting that she has to let go of her narcissistic desires before she can generously take care of her baby. But we all confront these issues at some time, and when we do, we have to face them honestly instead of feeling guilty about them. Only then can we move forward.

With the birth of my son, I became aware that my dreams of perfection had limits, and my vision of life's most precious event would have to be modified. I must have known then how beautiful he really was—as I know now how beautiful he always has been.

## Accommodating Loss

You may discover that some losses cut more deeply than others. If there are specific things you miss right now that weigh heavily on the definition you have of yourself, you should consider adjusting your life to restore them. Every woman must decide for herself what changes need to take priority. Women who find the lack of private time most frustrating can take steps to get help in the house to free themselves for some time alone. Women who are more affected by the change in their physical shape can try to get involved in an exercise program.

For many women, the temporary loss of career and the pending decision of when to return to work may require immediate attention. Most new mothers, regardless of their situation at home and regardless of whether or not they have PPD, will at some time struggle with the issue of working versus not working. Even if one of the options is not available due to extenuating circumstances, women will still describe intermittent feelings of ambivalence about their decision. Because the losses related to working or not working seem to affect so many women, both with and without PPD, we will examine this dilemma more closely.

## Returning to Work: Juggling Your Losses

The decision to work outside the home in the immediate postpartum period is almost always a very complex and painful one. Of course, sometimes it's not a decision at all, but a necessity. According to the US Bureau of the Census, one-half of all working women stay home for at least one year after the birth of a child. However, in these harsh economic times, more and more couples rely on the wife's income and simply cannot afford more than a brief maternity leave. Single mothers almost always have to go back to work right away.

Some mothers have no trouble deciding to return to work. They may never even consider the possibility of an extended maternity leave, because they love their jobs too much, are happy with their child care arrangements, or feel the professional consequences of staying home would be too costly. We also see a number of women who confess they would like to work part-time, but their husbands want them to stay home full-time.

Other women end up finding a middle ground. We have seen mothers who have been able to obtain job security after an extended leave of absence, who develop freelance jobs out of their homes, or who work in high-pressure jobs but only for two or three days per week.

We have not seen any single pattern of the effect of work on PPD. Some women tell us that returning to work helped alleviate the symptoms of PPD. Others have found that going to work seemed to make PPD worse, perhaps because work became just another place to fail or because of the stress of working, especially if it was out of necessity, not choice.

Whatever situation you are in with regard to work, there will most likely be some guilt or uncertainty associated with your decision. The following exercise can help you face these feelings and deal with them. If you are not currently employed outside of the home but were in the past, we encourage you to complete the following:

1. Think about how it used to feel to go to work. Describe your "old self" on a typical day at work. What did she look like?
2. How was her morning spent before work?
3. How was her time at work spent? What did she do?

4. What was the best part of her job?
5. What was the worst part of her job?
6. How did others see her?
7. How was her evening spent after work?
8. What do you miss most about her?

If you currently leave your baby at home with a sitter or at day care to go to work every day, complete the following:

1. What is the hardest part of the day for you?
2. How do you feel when you leave in the morning?
3. If you could stay home, what would your day be like?
4. How is work different and how do others treat you now that you have a baby at home?
5. How do you feel on your way home from work?
6. How do you spend your evening at home now?
7. What do you miss most about being on maternity leave?
8. How is going back to work different from being on leave?

There is no right or wrong answer to the question of going back to work. But we do have some ideas about how to make the choice and how to live with the decision you make. If for some reason working or not working outside the home is not an option, try to admit it and reconcile your situation. Valerie speaks from experience here:

As a resident in training, I had to go back to "call" (thirty-six-hour shifts in the hospital) when my first baby was only six weeks old. The medical profession has a strong ethic against "complaining" (that is to say, against acknowledging one's personal needs). I denied any emotional reaction I had to this state of affairs, thinking that I couldn't complain, because my patients and my colleagues needed me.

Instead of grieving the loss of the abrupt separation from my baby, I first denied it by trying to do it all. In between trips to the emergency room, you would find me expressing breast milk in the neonatal nursery or running around the hospital trying to find a freezer in which to store it. You can imagine the ultimate in role conflict: being paged while hooked up to an electric breast pump! I refused to admit that I was miserable and tried to be both perfect resident and perfect mother.

Fortunately, this didn't last too long. It became clear to me that I needed to ease up on both roles and let myself feel sad about working at such a hectic pace, even though I had chosen to have a baby during residency. When I admitted that this lifestyle was inherently stressful, I was able to let go of some of the self-inflicted stresses.

Yes, I did stop breastfeeding, and it was a very painful loss. I also had to let go of my wish to be a 100 percent available therapist, an ongoing struggle that surfaces whenever I need to limit my availability for meeting times or phone calls outside of therapy. As a strong supporter of equality in the workplace, I found it very difficult to acknowledge that I had special needs as a result of being a mother and felt as if I were a traitor to working women everywhere. Simply admitting that I was feeling losses allowed me to reach out for emotional support from people I trusted not to gloat over my inability to achieve superwoman status.

By contrast, Karen chose to stay home full-time for a longer period (one year with her first child, five months with her second) and to return on a part-time basis:

I was fortunate to have a job that gave me the option of returning to work after a year's maternity leave. So, right from the outset, I had a framework of security that I am convinced helped make my decision much less stressful. At that time in my life, I was willing to put career issues on hold while I spent time at home with my baby. This was before I had established my private practice, and since I was working in a hospital setting, I felt that my professional obligations and commitments were less personal and more bureaucratic.

I remember feeling quite ready to make taking care of my baby a priority. But all the preparation in the world could not possibly have alerted me to the reality of a twenty-four-hour schedule of new motherhood, one that challenged every ounce of my being. My instincts were good, and I trusted the choices I made. But every once in a while, when I wasn't looking, I got bitten by that bug of insecurity: "What if this isn't the right way to do this? Maybe I should have gone back to work, at least part-time. What if there's a better way?" It was often those very moments of doubt that forced me to take a second look at some of the choices I had made and thereby reinforce them.

When I went back to work, I recall struggling with my deep desire to return to my career and the pull I felt, gently tugging me back to my son. But I missed interacting with other adults, having people appreciate the work I was doing, having a place to go, and having a reason to put on grown-up clothes. And I knew the decision to return to work at that point was right for me.

No matter how much you want to go back to work, or how ready you think you are, there is no doubt that the day you actually do it ranks right up there as one of the most traumatic adaptations of new motherhood. It's hard to do when you've been home for a year. And it's hard to do when you've been home for three weeks. The conflict a woman endures when she must simultaneously care for her baby and herself doesn't ever go away completely—we just get a little better at dealing with it.

## To Work or Not to Work: Living with Ambivalence

Strangers, loved ones, colleagues, bosses, babysitters, grandmothers, and even therapists feel entitled to tell you whether or not you should go back to work. In our culture, mothers and babies are in the public domain, and therefore open to everybody's opinion and criticism.

Despite all this noise, try to listen to your own instincts about what is right for you, your baby, and your family.

Part of trusting your instincts involves accepting that ambivalence about the choice is natural. You are probably saying something like, "But everyone I know seems to love staying home with the baby!" or "Everyone I know seems to love working full-time!" We think they may just be better at hiding their own ambivalence. Whatever you decide, you will have days when you wish you could go to work or days when you would love to stay home. Ellen remembers how she used to gaze out her kitchen window as her neighbors would leave for work every morning. "I was jealous of every one of them. I wished so badly that I had some place I could go to get away for a little while. But inevitably, I would look at my sweet Katie and remind myself that I was doing the right thing for both of us. At least for now. Not a day would go by when I didn't wonder how it would feel to go back to work." Accepting your own ambivalence will help free you from judging yourself. You have made a choice for today and should expect to have some longings for life "on the other side."

While you are likely choking from good advice about whether or not to return to work, you may also find yourself right in the midst of a battle of values: "Mothers should stay home for at least a year in order to provide a consistent, nurturing environment for their growing child." Or, conversely, "Mothers who return to work before their child's first birthday experience a significant increase in self-esteem, which leads to more confident mothering, and report a higher degree of satisfaction with their chosen lifestyle." Depending on what you read or who you listen to, it can sound very confusing.

It is especially difficult if you are feeling pressure about this choice from someone close to you, like your husband or mother-in-law. Jennifer was two months postpartum when she remarked about her husband's position about her staying home, "It really surprised me to discover how traditional Tom was in some ways. When I told him I was thinking about going back to work part-time, he said he didn't want someone else raising our baby and that he wanted me to be home fulltime with our son. I was amazed by his attitude. Money was so tight; I thought he would want me to bring in another salary as soon as possible."

Conflicts of this nature need to be negotiated carefully. Something that may, at first glance, look like an issue on one level—like money or schedules—may in fact be related to larger issues such as the value of having a mother home on a full-time basis or the desire to reclaim your independence and self-esteem. We firmly believe that the most important concern is that you feel good about whatever decision you make. That will ultimately have the greatest impact on your growing child. Decisions are hard to make when you have PPD. Considering your choice as one that can be modified at a later time may help you to accept your decision. This is simply how you are managing this conflict now, not forever and ever.

## Reclaiming Your Self-Esteem

During this period of instability, you may feel as if you are abruptly being asked to redefine the essence of who you are: there are no more parties until 3 a.m., only wee-hour feedings. You can't impulsively do the crazy things you used to "just for fun," because you have skyrocketed into parenthood and must be a responsible role model twenty-four hours a day. You can't feel particularly sexy with sore nipples and breast milk leaking through your black lace nightgown. You are constantly being asked to adapt in ways you may have never thought possible. And before you can see how wonderful some of these changes may be, you must first feel the pain of each loss. Only then can you make your way beyond the sadness and welcome some of the new and positive feelings in store for you.

When you are depressed, persistent negative thoughts about yourself will damage self-esteem and lock you into a system of beliefs that wear away feelings of self-respect and, basically, liking yourself. As Cindy points out, "I can honestly say that I really didn't like myself when I had PPD. I didn't like what I thought about myself or how I thought about other people. Sometimes, I couldn't help it. But other times, I know it was just a whole lot easier to feel bad about myself."

Although it may be tempting to dwell on the negative aspects of your life, why not try to use some of that energy toward rebuilding a positive image of yourself. Think about the following questions in an effort to focus on areas of your life that actually feel good to you right now. (If you can't think of an answer to one of these questions, skip it and go on. If you skip more than three, it may be premature to attempt this, and we suggest you put aside this exercise until you are feeling better.)

1. What is one thing you find pleasure in doing now?

   _____

2. What are you looking forward to in the immediate future?

   _____

3. What are you looking forward to in the distant future?

   _____

4. What is the best part about having this baby?

   _____

5. In what way do you surpass your expectations of yourself as mother?

   _____

6. What have you gotten better at since the birth of your baby?

   _____

7. Do you continue to do the things you did before you had the baby that made you feel good about yourself? If not, why not?

   _____

8. List four qualities you have that you like:

   _____

   _____

_____

_____

9. List four qualities you have that others like:

_____

_____

_____

_____

Are you surprised at how many good things you could think about yourself? It is important for you to understand that you have not lost your "old self" forever. You are responding to the physical, hormonal, psychological, biochemical, and emotional demands of this transitional time. As in any crisis, we learn to respond and behave in new ways by drawing on available resources.

Once you begin to feel better about yourself—which will be in part due to your deliberate efforts, and in part due to the course of PPD and eventual symptom relief—you will feel more equipped to take responsibility for controlling your own life and accept the uncertainties that are a natural part of this passage into motherhood.

The parts of yourself that seem far out of reach right now have only taken a temporary leave of absence to provide you with room to develop new skills, new feelings, and new parts of yourself. When you accept your losses, you open up possibilities that allow you to take better care of yourself, such as requesting and accepting emotional support from someone you trust. Later on, as you continue to recover, reminders of your old self will trickle back in and reposition themselves. Eventually, everything will begin to integrate, and you will feel more together.

# ·ᐂ[ 13 ]ᐂ·

# "WILL I BE JUST LIKE MY MOTHER?"

## Working Through Intergenerational Issues

*Marcie inspected herself in the mirror. She looked tired and drawn. As she gently wiped the moisturizer into her cheeks, she heard her oldest child bullying his baby sister. Marcie sighed. Not sure whether she could make it through another day like yesterday, she turned abruptly and yelled, "If you two don't stop this nonsense right now, you will both spend all day in your rooms!" She turned back to the mirror, looked straight into her own wide eyes, and said softly to herself, "Oh, my God . . . I'm turning into my mother!"*

SOMETIMES, THE WORDS SOUND exactly the same. Other times, it's not what you say, but how you say it that reminds you of your mother. Many women find humor in this identification. Other women find it disquieting and worrisome.

When a woman becomes pregnant and gives birth to a child, she often notices herself being drawn to her own mother. Often, this is the first opportunity she has had to identify so completely with the statements, thoughts, and actions of the woman who raised her. Words that were often resented or ignored can now be appreciated with new understanding. The challenge of this introspective journey can be quite rewarding to some women, as it offers an opportunity for new dialogue between mother and daughter.

Other women, with or without PPD, discover that the birth of a child throws them into a crisis* with their own mothers. The crisis emerges as a result of the contradiction between your often powerful residual need to be mothered and your commitment to be a strong, independent, and yes, perfect mother to your own child. Although the need to be "mothered" right now may seem regressive, if not ridiculous, most women who are honest with themselves do get in touch with some primitive desires to be taken care of during the first months after having a baby. Some women can readily admit their desire to be fed, nurtured, held, and pampered during this time. Yet, while these feelings are very strong, they are often opposed by equally powerful urges to separate completely and function independently.

Having a baby may trigger a variety of conflicting feelings about your relationship with your mother. When you have PPD, you may find yourself needing her more than ever, and resenting what you perceive as your own weakness. You may find that the more you try to pull away from your mother, the more you need her.

Perhaps something she does or says that you used to be able to tolerate or ignore suddenly hurts you deeply. Whatever the dynamics are for you, one thing is certain: this can be a wonderful opportunity for mothers and daughters to address some of the old, often suppressed issues that surface during this time and to begin to relate as adults.

---

* When we refer to this crisis in a woman's life, we are talking about a normal developmental crisis within a woman's search for identity. This chapter is not designed to help you come to grips with a lifelong abusive, neglectful, or otherwise seriously problematic relationship with your mother. If this is the case for you, it will make you feel worse to do the work in this chapter; these issues and feelings need to be discussed with a therapist.

Women with PPD will often benefit tremendously by exploring their relationship with their mothers, although this process may involve a great deal of ambivalence and conflict, with an associated anxiety.

Our understanding of the role our fathers play in the development of our expectations and life choices is much less clear. This is not to suggest that his role is less significant than our mothers. However, adults cannot help but look to their same-sex parents for role modeling at major life transition points such as marriage and childbirth.

While unresolved issues with your parents are not the cause of your PPD, because the illness has lowered your resistance and increased your emotional vulnerabilities, everything becomes magnified. And although your reactions may seem way out of proportion and somewhat out of your control, now is actually a good time to take a closer look at your parental relationships in order to understand the effect they have had on your life.

The exercises in this chapter are very specific and require you to draw upon some detailed memories of your relationship with your mother. If this is painful, you need to determine whether it would be better for you to put this aside, enlist the help of a professional, or push ahead.

If your mother is no longer living, this chapter will probably have particular resonance for you. Most women who have suffered the loss of their mother find childbirth especially poignant. The juxtaposition of life and death, ecstasy and grief, can set off a whirlwind of emotions. If you factor in the additional losses experienced by a woman with PPD, the sadness is greatly compounded. Ellen, who we introduced in the last chapter, recalls how she felt. "I wanted my mother to have been able to see my baby. I cried for days after he was born. I felt so happy and so sad at the same time. I loved my baby and I missed my mom so. I just wish she could have held him once."

If you have lost your mother, try to think about some of the questions in this chapter as they relate to the relationship you had with her when she was alive. She is still very much a part of your life, and your identification with her is just as strong as it was before she died.

The purpose of this chapter is to help you understand that working through some of the issues you have with your mother—both old, unresolved ones from childhood and new ones—will have a direct impact on how you feel about yourself as a mother. For this reason, we will explore the mother-daughter relationship from your childhood as well as the one you have now. After we identify and work through some of the pressing concerns, we will explore the concept of forgiving our mothers and letting go of old pain.

## Identification with Your Mother

Identification refers to the act or process of becoming like someone else by internalizing (usually unconsciously) both positive and negative parts of that person. People with whom we identify usually have influenced us in very direct and meaningful ways, like our mothers.

As you recall some of these details about your mother and your relationship with her, you may begin to get in touch with some of the hurt you have locked away. If you do, remember that our goal here is to work toward reconciliation with your mother and these feelings so you can feel better about yourself, not to set off a cycle of blame and revenge. Women with PPD and women without PPD will struggle through this. Women who have good, solid relationships with their mothers and women who have ongoing battles with their mothers will find this work difficult. Try to remember that the pain will end, and that unless you go through the pain of confronting these issues, they will continue to haunt you and delay your recovery.

When you were pregnant, you might have noticed that there were times when you began fantasizing about the kind of mother you were going to be. Many of these fantasies were directly related to how you felt about the way your own mother took care of you. What kind of mother was she?

◉ Was she nurturing and compassionate?

◉ Was she cold and strict?

◉ Did she take the time to explain things to you?

◉ Did she encourage you to think for yourself?

◉ Did she overprotect you?

◉ Did she make you feel important? Attractive?

◉ Did she keep you safe?

## Descriptive Identification: What She Did

Understanding your mother in descriptive terms will help you define the parameters of your idealized self as mother. In other words, recalling what your mother was like will enable you to understand further the ways that you have identified with her, both positively and negatively. Because so much of this identification is unconscious, you may be unaware of how similar you really are until you focus on particulars.

List five things about you that are just like your mother:

*Examples:* I clean my house every opportunity I get.

I am very emotional.

1. _____
2. _____
3. _____
4. _____
5. _____

List five ways in which you are different from your mother:

*Examples:* I set fewer restrictions on my child's behavior.

I didn't choose to return to work after my baby was born.

1. _____
2. _____

3. _____
4. _____
5. _____

How do you feel about these similarities and differences? Go back over the lists and indicate which you are comfortable with and which are troublesome for you. Think about why you feel that way. Ellen tells this story about her mother:

> I remember my mother always doing everything for everyone. No matter who it was or what they wanted, she would take care of it. When I was young, I used to think she was a miracle mom, always fixing everything. Then, as I got older, I realized all of those good deeds were taking her away from me, and she never had time for herself. As I grew up, I resented the "good things" she did for everyone else. Now, I find that I'm doing the exact same thing! My husband said to me the other night, "Could you just stop for five minutes and sit with me?" I wasn't even aware that I was running around the way she always did. I wonder why I do that.

In what specific ways would you like to repeat your mother's pattern of mothering?

1. _____
2. _____
3. _____

In what specific ways do you hope to differ from your mother's style of child rearing?

1. _____
2. _____
3. _____

Sometimes, your perceptions of what your mother was doing and how or why she did it were way off base. Consider Marcie as she sits in a therapy session along with her mother:

> I remember my mother as the most calm, cool, collected, capable woman. She cooked and cleaned and took care of all four of us and still managed to look perfect and beautiful. After a day of trying to hold my life together, I look in the mirror at my disheveled appearance, flop on the unmade bed, think about the difference between us, and feel like a complete failure!

Her mom responded with a tear in her eye.

> I don't know whose house you were living in! I was a complete wreck most of the time. Dr. Peters had me on Valium; otherwise, I wouldn't have slept a wink! I guess all I was good at was fooling you kids into thinking I knew what I was doing.

Taking the time to evaluate your mother's mothering will enable you to get a clearer picture of what you value most in your own maternal endeavors. Also, thinking about these comparisons now will significantly reduce the likelihood that you will be concerned about them later, which would make you feel worse.

## Emotional Identification: How She Made You Feel

Sometimes, how we feel about ourselves and how we respond emotionally to others is related to our emotional connection with our primary caretaker. If you take a closer look at your mother, you may learn some interesting things about yourself. When completing the following statements, try to recall when you were younger and focus on that time. Describe your mother in terms of her capacity to meet your emotional needs and how it feels now to remember it.

1.  One of the things my mother was always best at was

    _____

    This makes me feel

    _____

2.  When I was sad, my mother would

    _____

    This makes me feel

    _____

3.  It was easy/hard to talk to my mother because

    _____

    This makes me feel

    _____

4.  One of the ways my mother made me feel important was

    _____

    This makes me feel

    _____

5.  My favorite thing to do with my mother was

    _____

    This makes me feel

    _____

6.  My mother loved it when I used to

    _____

    This makes me feel

    _____

7.  I knew I could please my mother if I would

    _____

    This makes me feel

    _____

8.  When I was scared, my mother would

    _____

    This makes me feel

    _____

9. If I could have said something to my mother as a child that could have changed things, I would have told her

_____

This makes me feel

_____

10. I often wished that my mother was able to

_____

This makes me feel

_____

11. It made me so angry that my mother never/always

_____

This makes me feel

_____

12. I will never forget my mother telling me

_____

This makes me feel

_____

As you become more critical of some of the choices your mother made or some of the things she did, you will find yourself experiencing a variety of feelings associated with these memories. For instance, look at number 8, "When I was scared, my mother would tell me I wasn't being a big girl and I should grow up. Now, that makes me sad and angry. Wouldn't it have been great if she had told me it was okay to be scared? And maybe told me what I could do when I felt that way?"

As you complete these exercises, keep in mind that you are not trying to blame your mother for anything. What you are doing is trying to increase your understanding of how she influenced you in order to learn more about yourself.

Since having your baby, you may feel as though you are in a much better position to review some of the choices made by your mother and to make some generalizations about the way you want to raise your child. Some of your mother's choices were "good" choices (ones that seemed to have been in your best interest; choices that you might make today), and others were "bad" choices (those that perhaps did not work toward your own best interest; choices that you would not make today). But unless you analyze the effects your mother's choices had on you, you may not be able to distinguish between the two and may end up either inflicting the same emotional wounds you suffered on your child or missing opportunities to bolster his strengths.

## How Am I Doing, Mom?

Most women never completely outgrow the need for approval from their mothers. It seems that no matter how old we get or how grown up we like to think we are, most of us can admit that it always feels good to hear our mothers tell us we're doing a great job. Some women may never have heard that growing up, so they long for it now—their mothers' expectations were so high that no matter how good a job they did, it was never enough. Other women may have been so overprotected and indulged that they have a hard time discriminating whether they have done something right or wrong.

More than one woman has confessed to us that she secretly wishes her mother could look over her shoulder during the 3 a.m. feeding and sweetly whisper, "You must be so tired. You are doing such a wonderful job. I'm so proud of you. You are such a good mother."

If you have gotten that message from your mother, you know how good her approval feels. If you have not, you are probably still aching for it. Try telling those same words to yourself. It is difficult, but it is possible for you to mother yourself. If it's not likely that you will get nurturing from anyone else, you must learn to give it to yourself.

Think about these questions:

- How important is it to you that your mother thinks you are doing a good job right now?

* Do you want and/or need her approval?
* How much influence does she have on the way you feel about yourself in your new role as mother?

There are no right answers to any of the questions in this chapter, nor will what you do with this information after you think about it be the same as any other new mother. But for most women with PPD, this difficult journey back home to their mothers can offer comfort and new insight into the transition to motherhood. If, on the other hand, you experience any disturbing response as you read this chapter, it is time to put it away. If you are in therapy, this is a good chapter to work through with your therapist, so she can help you sort these feelings out and keep them in perspective.

## Dynamic Identification:
## Your Mother Today

Many women are surprised to discover how much their present relationship with their own mother, whether amicable or stressful, determines how they will feel about themselves as a mother. Your current relationship with your mother seems to carry a great deal of weight when evaluating the expectations you have as well as the accomplishments you have made. Understanding this relationship can help you feel more confident about your own mothering skills.

Think about how you feel about your relationship with your mother today:

1.  What I respect most about my mother is

    _____

2.  What I dislike most about my mother is

    _____

3.  My mother is most helpful when she

    _____

4.  If I could change one thing about my relationship with my
    mother, it would be

    _____

5.  The way my mother feels about my baby is

    _____

6.  What I love most about my mother is

    _____

8.  I feel hurt when my mother

    _____

9.  Since I have become a mother, my relationship with my mother
    has changed in that

    _____

10. If my mother were to describe me as a mother, she would
    say

    _____

As you complete these statements, note again how each one makes
you feel. Your answers may trigger feelings that range from resentment, anger, and frustration to comfort, contentment, and love. All of
these feelings are okay.

Focusing on your relationship with your mother at this time can
be difficult, because it forces you to alternate between your accus-
tomed role as child and your new role as parent. Because the transition is so recent, this duality may be very interesting. You may feel as
though you are being forced to grow up, and that can be very scary
and exciting at the same time.

## Understanding Your Mother

Remember Marcie, who was stunned by her seemingly abrupt trans-
formation into her mother?

Marcie was standing in the kitchen trying to get dinner ready one night, listening to her children. One was screaming from her high chair asking for one thing, the other was "needing" her to do something else. Dinner was burning, and the work she planned to do around the house had not gotten done. She paused for a moment and realized, perhaps for the first time, what her own mother must have gone through raising her and her sisters. It dawned on her that her mother was not just her mother, but a woman, a wife, a person with desires, needs, other responsibilities, hobbies, deadlines, constraints, and various distractions. Marcie realized that she still harbored a vision of this all-powerful mother who existed only to meet the needs of her children. It was a bittersweet recognition for Marcie, and it enabled her to reach out to her mother on a level that she had not previously been able to do.

Many women, like Marcie, discover that becoming a parent gives them a second chance at building a strong relationship with their mother. It allows them the opportunity to relate to each other as equals, in a way that was not previously possible. One way for you to secure this new perspective is to find out about the parts of your mother's life that have nothing to do with you. How well do you know your mother? Try to answer the following questions about her. If you do not know the answer, or find that you are interested in more information from her, you should plan a special time to get together and talk.

1. To the best of your knowledge, what events in your mother's childhood significantly affected who she was and how she felt about herself? (*Examples*: death of a loved one, divorce, medical illness, alcoholism, abuse, violence, abandonment)

   _____

2. What kind of a role model did your mother have for her mothering practices?

   _____

3. What circumstances, if any, made it particularly difficult for her to be a mother during the time when you were a child?

_____

4. What kind of support did your mother have from your father? What role did he play in raising the children?

_____

5. What values were most important to your mother? Why were they so important to her?

_____

6. Did your mother enjoy being a mother?

_____

## Communicating with Your Mother

Many women find it interesting and quite comforting to explore some of the issues raised in this chapter with their mothers. This is a decision you should consider carefully. Obviously, you will be the best judge of whether or not your relationship will benefit from this sort of confrontation, especially if most of the feelings you have gotten in touch with are negative ones. On the other hand, if you and your mother have always been able to express yourselves openly to each other, you may be eager to share what you have learned.

If such a confrontation feels overwhelming to you right now, put that suggestion aside. You will still benefit from your self-disclosure alone. For the time being, why don't you organize some of your thoughts in the form of a letter? Even though this letter is not intended to be mailed, writing it is a good way of getting some of your ideas out in a nonthreatening, nonconfrontational way.

Here is a sample letter:

Dear Mom,

I wish you could understand what I am going through. I know you always tried to do your best. Right now, I just need you to listen to me and tell me that everything is going to be okay. Sometimes I am really scared. And I'm afraid to tell you, because then you'll think I'm not a good mother. I'm so scared you will think that. I am doing my best right now, just like you did. I just need to know it's all right for me to fail sometimes.

I mean, as long as everyone is safe and protected. I need to know that I can make a mistake. It's no big deal, right? Please tell me everything will be okay. I love you.

Love, Jane

Dear Mom,

_____

_____

_____

_____

_____

_____

_____

Love,

_____

## Forgiving Your Mother

Your relationship with your mother is perhaps the most influential connection you will ever have in your life. Within every mother-child bond there exist conflicting elements of unconditional love, support, nurturance, intimacy, separation, deprivation, overprotection, and abandonment. And though we have all fantasized about that storybook mother who can answer all our questions, soothe all our fears, make all of our pain go away, and who exists only to meet our every need, we know she is only make-believe. Those of us who have been trying to be good mothers for a while now continue to discover our own limitations and failures. No matter how desperately we try to do everything "right," we are soon confronted by our own imperfect efforts and rely on the hope that our children will understand that we did the best we could and ultimately forgive us.

Your mother also did the best she could. And although our dream of the perfect mother may persist, the greatest gift we can give ourselves and our mothers is the understanding that compromise and acceptance can pave the way for new directions and better relationships. When we forgive our mothers for the mistakes they made, we let go of the anger and resentment that gets in the way of genuine emotional connections. The act of forgiving does not mean you agree with what was done or said. It means you will not hold your mother responsible for your negative feelings anymore. It means you will choose either to build a new bond, one that will grow and develop as you evolve through motherhood, or to recognize that this simply isn't possible and let go.

If your mother is not living or if you have lost touch with her, it is still possible to reach deep within your sadness and to come to terms with your past relationship. We urge you to do this.

## Your Relationship with Your Father

In many ways, a woman's self-esteem is linked to her relationship with her father and how successful he was at communicating his feelings to her. Many women complain that their father was not as available as they would have liked. This was often due to social and financial pressures and cultural conventions. Although this may be understood on an intellectual level, many women admit that they continue to seek approval and acceptance from their fathers throughout their adult lives. Spend some time thinking about your relationship with your father:

- Did your parents have an intact marriage throughout the years you lived at home with them?

- How would you describe the relationship between your father and mother?
- Can you describe a typical daily routine with your dad when you were young? (For example: breakfast with Mom and Dad, Dad leaves for work, Dad not home for dinner, Dad home when we were in bed, never saw him on weekends because he worked, etc.)
- What was your favorite thing to do with your dad?
- What did you need from your father then?
- What do you need from your father now?
- In what ways are you like your father that feel good to you?
- In what ways are you like your father that do not feel good to you?
- Do you remember your father holding you, hugging you, telling you he loved you?
- If you could say anything at all to your father, what would you like to ask of him today?

As you think about these questions, be aware of your emotional response. You may find yourself feeling angry at your dad or perhaps sad about days gone by. You may miss his comfort and support, or you may wonder where he has been when you needed him. This exercise helps get you in touch with some of the early-childhood feelings you may have buried that could still be affecting your relationship with your father. Sometimes, it is enough just to feel them—nothing else needs to be done. Some women, on the other hand, use this opportunity to talk to their fathers in ways similar to those described for their mothers: gentle confrontation, a letter-writing exercise, or simply a face-to-face exchange of feelings and information.

As you look over the work you have done to uncover these feelings that relate to your mother and father in this chapter, remember that we are not implying that these issues with your parents have caused PPD. If, however, you suspect that the issues raised here were, indeed, major factors in the emergence of PPD, then we hope you are addressing these subjects in therapy. Furthermore, if you feel that the work you have started here is not enough, we urge you to continue your exploration with a professional. Remember that human inter-actions are dynamic. As your PPD symptoms begin to resolve, and as you continue to build on the work you have started here, you may be rewarded by seeing some positive changes in these primary relation-ships. It is definitely worth the effort.

# "I'M STARTING TO FEEL LIKE MYSELF AGAIN"

## As You Begin to Recover

*I felt so good yesterday, like my old self again. It was wonderful. I thought for sure I was better. Now I feel funny again. Why is this happening?*

—HEATHER, IN THERAPY SIX MONTHS POSTPARTUM

RECOVERY IS AN ONGOING PROCESS with a beginning, middle, and end. While the specific course of recovery differs for each individual, there are certain features that are fairly typical of the recovery period. As we discuss these phases, keep in mind that these are descriptive guidelines that will not apply to every woman in the same way.

# Phases of Recovery

### Early Recovery

You may begin to notice that other people think you're better before you do. This is common. Chances are, you're getting pretty good at putting on a cheerful face for the world, and soon you will hear comments like, "I see you're back to your old self again!" or the equally insensitive, albeit well-meaning, "See, having a baby isn't so bad, is it?"

Although this kind of feedback may feel a bit premature, other people may have a more objective perspective that allows them to pick up signs of improvement before you do. When you hear comments that suggest you may be beginning to recover, try to see them as anticipatory and, most likely, reliable measures of this first phase of the recovery process. If you find such comments to be bothersome, there are several ways you can respond to statements like, "You look wonderful. You must be feeling great."

1. You can ignore them.
2. You can refocus by acknowledging what was said, but adding a piece of reality, such as "Yes, I'm starting to have good days now."
3. You can deflect them by saying, "Thank you," or some other vague comment.

We find there are three features that characterize this early stage of recovery: *Doubt, Distraction,* and *Rediscovery.*

As Heather left her therapist's office, she was relieved to hear that she was getting better and that all her hard work was paying off. Heather took a deep breath and stood up straight as she walked out the door, feeling for the first time in a long while that she might actually be getting back on track. But then she started wondering if she had misheard the therapist. Maybe she wasn't doing as well as she thought. Maybe she had just convinced her therapist that things looked good, but inside, nothing had really changed. "What about that bad day I had last week? I forgot to mention that to her. If she knew how bad I felt that day, I'm sure she wouldn't think I was doing so well."

These feelings of *doubt* are central to this early phase and will not impede recovery. Although they may discourage you intermittently, do not misinterpret them as a sign of regression. They indicate a normal phase of the process of recovery. It's perfectly understandable that with so much at stake, you will have moments of uncertainty.

As you begin to feel better, you may notice that you are thinking less about the way you feel. *Distraction* seems to be one of the most common characteristics of this early stage of recovery.

Heather describes it like this:

It's like I have to think about the fact that I'm not thinking about PPD so much. It's not the first thing I think about anymore. Before, as soon as I opened my eyes in the morning, my brain would start working, asking myself: How do I feel? How bad is it today? Oh no, I felt this way yesterday. Now, I awake, get up, get dressed, and I'm halfway down the stairs before I realize, hey—I don't feel so terrible this morning.

During this period of distraction, there is a tendency to refocus your attention from yourself to something external, such as other people, work, or hobbies. You may find yourself rediscovering some of the simple things that used to provide pleasure, such as calling friends on the phone, gardening, or relaxing with a good book. When this occurs, it often brings enormous relief from the constant ruminations and cycles of despair that dominated your way of thinking while you were in the throes of PPD.

*Rediscovery* of previously pleasurable activities and feelings provides many women with the first real sign that they are headed in the right direction. When you are able to retrieve familiar, comfortable feelings that were shut out during the acute phases of PPD, you will begin to feel more like yourself.

Heather remembers how good it felt when she went to the mall for the first time since she had been in therapy.

> I know it sounds silly, but something just kept me from going there when I felt bad. There were too many people. I always thought they were looking at me, as if somehow they would see what a failure I was. I forgot how much I missed going, until I went back for the first time. It was great! I felt like a kid in a candy store. I didn't know where to go first. I knew this was a good sign.

## MIDDLE RECOVERY

The middle phase of recovery is distinguished by its unstable and often unpredictable nature and is often referred to as the roller coaster phase.

Heather described this pattern to her therapist.

> Sometimes I feel like I'm on a roller coaster. I feel great for five days. (See, I know I'm not completely better, because I'm still counting the number of days!) Then, I feel terrible. But it doesn't last long, and all of a sudden, I feel good again. I feel like I'm going in circles. It's definitely better than before. In fact, sometimes I think I'm completely better, then, wham! A bad day comes out of nowhere.

This fluctuation of moods can be quite distressing during a time when you are just beginning to feel back in control. The good days feel terrific, and the bad days make you feel like you're back at square one. It should reassure you to know that these mood variations are characteristic of the middle recovery phase and are not indicative of a long-term setback, but rather a sign that recovery is in full swing. Intermittent feelings of depression and sadness are common during this time. So are feelings of renewed hope and optimism. This is not a time to abandon the lessons and coping skills you have learned. It is time to gain control as you balance the bad days with the good ones that are around the corner.

During this phase of recovery, some women experience a surge of energy they describe as exhilarating. Although this can feel wonderful, caution is advised. This is when many women make the mistake of overexerting themselves. We recommend using this new energy in areas of relationships and play only: spend time with your baby, go to the beach or pool, visit a friend, have lunch with your husband. Do not use this energy to throw a Tupperware party, do spring cleaning, or paint the baby's room. If you do, you may take a step backward. Some women insist that they have to find this out for themselves, and they continue to push their limits. Trust us. We've seen it happen many times in our practices. If you overextend yourself, you can get worse. The energy feels good now, but if you burn it all up, you will be left with fatigue, which likely played a strong contributing role in the development of your PPD in the first place. You should not put yourself at risk for increased fatigue until you have fully recovered.

## LATE RECOVERY

The final stage of recovery involves periods of readjustment and reflection. During the period of readjustment, women are faced with the challenge of finding a new equilibrium as a result of their recent PPD crisis. Reestablishing a routine after being uprooted so abruptly requires a system of ongoing accommodations.

Heather expressed caution during this phase and appeared quite tentative in her efforts to adjust to all of the changes in her life.

I feel pretty good lately. I'm afraid to say I feel great, 'cause I'm not sure how long this will last. Yesterday, I talked to my boss about going back to work part-time. It feels good to be ready to tackle the world again. But sometimes I wonder if it will be too much for me. How do I know when I'm really ready, when I am over my PPD?

The most difficult challenge of this phase is the successful integration of your new perception of yourself. All the self-help work you have been doing has heightened your awareness of parts of yourself that were previously unknown. As you have discovered, sometimes these perceptions are not the most positive. For instance, you might now be aware that anxiety attacks are often how you respond to stress. And although you have learned to temper that response, to expect the total absence of these attacks would be unrealistic at this point. This is why we say that part of the readjusting that you will be doing is accepting that some of these changes will continue to be a part of your life right now. Some of the symptoms that were so intrusive earlier can now be viewed as limitations. There is nothing wrong with limitations, like mild anxiety or an occasional sleepless night. The key is to deal with them in such a way that you can still enjoy the good things in your life. That is what you are learning to do in this final stage of the recovery process.

After you gain a little confidence that some of these new good feelings will last, you may notice that you begin to reflect on the progress you have made and the general effect PPD has had on you. As you continue to feel stronger and more like yourself, you may notice that you become almost driven to find answers to this whole episode. Many women note that they continue to think about PPD, but from a broader perspective than when they were in the most acute phase of the illness. They reflect on the overall impact PPD has had on various aspects of their lives and specifically on their marriages and relationships with their babies.

PPD causes a great strain on many marriages. Periods of readjustment may include waves of instability and conflict, particularly if the recovery process is rushed by either partner. Marital issues that have been put on hold during the course of the depression may surface all at once, endangering the effort to get things back on track. Couples who are aware that this latent pressure on their marriage is a natural part of this process are much more likely to be prepared for this transition. If you are in therapy, and if your husband has played an active role throughout your recovery, this is an important time to include him in your therapy in order to reinforce the strengths in your marriage and address any areas of concern.

As you continue to recover and resume normal activities, an interesting phenomenon may occur. You may find that your husband begins to decompensate. As you get stronger, the equilibrium of the relationship often shifts, and your husband may relax his hold on whatever psychological resources helped get him through this crisis. Though he, too, was overwhelmed, he may have suppressed these feelings. It's as if when you needed oxygen, he held his breath, but now he needs extra air. As you get stronger, he may begin to let some of these feelings surface and may become disillusioned, exhausted, irritable, or depressed. When this occurs, women often respond with confusion and anger: "I'm finally feeling better, and now you fall apart?"

If you find that your husband is experiencing any of these negative feelings on a regular basis, you need to address this with him seriously. Talk it over and reassure him that you still need his support and that you feel strong enough to support him, also. On a good day, do something just for him: make his favorite dinner or get a sitter and go to the movie of his choice. This juxtaposition of feelings often remits spontaneously, and although professional support for your husband should always be an option, intervention is usually not necessary beyond your understanding and ongoing dialogue with him.

## Questions About Recovery

At this point in recovery, it is important to address resuming a sexual relationship. If you haven't done so yet, you need to begin talking about your feelings about your sexuality with your husband. He may expect your libido to return early in recovery, while it may actually be one of the last things to return.

### MEDICATION AND RECOVERY

When an antidepressant has been prescribed, recovery may appear to happen all at once. As one woman said, "I swear, at two o'clock yesterday afternoon—exactly twenty-one days and seventeen hours after we started the medication—it kicked in. All of a sudden, I had energy and enthusiasm again. I took my four-year-old out for pizza for the first time since the baby was born. I even did laundry and wrote a few thank-you notes."

This instantaneous recovery is extremely electrifying, and the temptation to rush back into a full schedule of activities is great. We encourage you to take it easy though, for the reasons described in the previous section on recovery. Overextending yourself increases the risk of a minor setback.

Not all women taking medication experience the kind of recovery often described as, "The dark cloud just seemed to lift." For many, recovery is much more gradual, with stops and starts, as described in the section above.

### WHAT IS THE RISK OF RELAPSE? CAN THIS HAPPEN WITHOUT HAVING ANOTHER BABY?

Concerns about a relapse or recurrence are common throughout recovery. Relapse refers to active return of symptoms after a remission has been induced; recurrence is a separate illness episode in the future. We will address these risks separately for those who recovered with medication versus those in psychotherapy or women relying on self-help.

We divide recovery into these two groups because, in general, those who needed and responded to medication had more severe forms of PPD than those who recovered using self-help and/or professional psychotherapy alone. The more severe your PPD, the greater the risk of relapse or recurrence.

If antidepressant medication played a significant role in your recovery, you may be wondering whether you should stop it once you feel better. Since the risk of relapse is highest in the first few months after medication is started, we almost always recommend continuing medication for six to twelve months after a noticeable improvement. A general guideline is to stay on an antidepressant medication through the first postpartum year, since it is so stressful, but this should be discussed with your doctor.

The risk of recurrence is much higher if this episode of PPD is not the first time you have suffered from depression, panic disorder, or obsessive-compulsive disorder. If you have a history of one or more previous episodes of clinical depression or anxiety, your doctor may recommend staying on antidepressant medication indefinitely, or you yourself may request that.

> Stephanie had her first child at age thirty-seven, with a severe case of PPD soon after. In retrospect, she recalled having two similar episodes, one in her late teens when she started college, and one at age thirty-one, for no apparent reason. Even though the depressions were far apart, it seemed that each was worse than the one before. When her psychiatrist told her that long-term maintenance medication was likely to prevent further episodes, Stephanie opted to stay on her antidepressant "forever," or at least until she decided whether she wanted to have another baby.

There is growing concern among mental-health professionals that individuals with moderate to severe recurrent depression may get worse symptoms or harder-to-treat illnesses with each subsequent episode of depression. This is another reason to consider long-term medication if this is not your first episode. However, no one knows whether a woman whose depressions have occurred only in the postpartum setting is at risk for clinical depression in general, so we hesitate to recommend indefinite medication in that case.

Longer-term medication maintenance may also be recommended after a single episode of PPD if your symptoms reappear when the medication is tapered. At the end of the period of time that you and your doctor decide—most likely the six to twelve months mentioned above—your medication dose should be very gradually lowered until it is discontinued. You should never stop your medication abruptly, because you will likely get some rebound or withdrawal symptoms that may cause the false perception that you still need the medication. However, relapsing symptoms that occur during or after a slow tapering generally do mean that you should continue at a full-maintenance dose before trying to go off again in four to six months.

It is also a good idea to taper gradually either psychotherapy or a program of self-help, in order to help prevent a relapse in the first six to twelve months. We recommend maintenance psychotherapy for several months after a remission has occurred. For example, if you met with your therapist weekly for three months until you were completely recovered, we suggest follow-up appointments every four to six weeks for the first postpartum year. Likewise, if the part of this book that really seemed to help was the section on developing social support, be sure not to retreat into your home the minute you get well. Instead, continue these efforts to reach out to others and maintain an active social network. The same applies to whatever aspect of this book helped you recover.

Unlike medication, psychotherapy and/or self-help don't leave your system once you stop them. If they have helped you develop better coping skills or self-esteem, you are more likely to be able to continue to call on these resources at times of future crises. Keep in mind that old habits die hard, so you may need "booster" sessions and should not view it as a failure if you occasionally need to consult a psychotherapist again. Those who developed postpartum stress syndrome are at higher risk for recurrences at other times of extreme stress in their lives. Longer-term psychotherapy (up to one or two years, typically) can help you make the kinds of psychological changes that increase your resistance to depression, anxiety, and stress or adjustment disorders.

## FURTHER CONSIDERATIONS

We've tried to address as many facets of the PPD experience as possible. Here are additional questions women in our practices have asked us.

### *"How will PPD affect my baby?"*

There are some worrisome studies indicating that a severely depressed woman does not interact with her infant in the same way she does when she is recovered. We don't know that there are any long-term consequences, but it does tell us two things: 1) it is very important to get well and do whatever you have to do to remedy your PPD, and 2) you should make every effort to have somebody who feels well help care for your baby during the time you are in crisis. After the PPD is over, some women feel guilty because they had to leave their babies with alternative caretakers (grandmother, father, aunt, babysitter). But it was important and actually good for the baby to be exposed to other caretakers who could consistently interact with a smile.

### *"Since I know I'm at risk for PPD, is there anything I can do to reduce the likelihood of a full-blown crisis after a future pregnancy?"*

Clinical evidence shows us that a previous postpartum depression does place a woman at higher risk for PPD in the future. Although we cannot specify your individual risk, we can state some generalities. The same features of PPD that are used to predict a response to medication also predict a greater likelihood of recurrence. These include major sleep and appetite changes, severity of symptoms, strong family predisposition, and early onset in the postpartum period. Suicidal thoughts, presence of psychosis, marked agitation, and the need for hospitalization also suggest a higher risk of recurrence.

We are often asked to help a woman predict her individual risk of recurrence. It is purely a judgment call, since no one can know with certainty. However, it is a good idea to anticipate the possibility of a recurrence, as it will allow you to develop a "what if" plan from a position of strength rather than in a time of weakness. Some women decide to maximize support from others and actively plan to nurture themselves in an attempt to minimize the postpartum stress that can trigger depression. Other women decide to begin medication late in pregnancy (in severe cases), or (more commonly) immediately after delivery as a preventive measure. Still others may feel more comfortable just knowing that they have a supportive therapist and/or doctor lined up "just in case."

The good news is that some women who do experience a second PPD report significantly less distress due to their increased awareness and anticipation of some of the symptoms. It does make a difference to detect and begin treatment right away, as was seen in the doctor's story in Chapter 10. Early intervention will augment your recovery, and anything you can do to prepare for the possibility of PPD recurring will strengthen your ability to adjust to it.[*]

Here is a list of things you can do to decrease the likelihood or the impact of recurrent PPD:

1. Explore your feelings about impending motherhood and share them with your husband. Discuss how you both feel about having another child and what your expectations are of each other.

---

[*] Karen explores this issue in depth in her book, *What Am I Thinking? Having a Baby After Postpartum Depression*.

2. Take good care of your physical self.
   - Get plenty of rest
   - Eat nutritious meals and snacks
   - Pamper yourself whenever possible
   - Exercise

3. Make preparations for help in the home after the baby comes. Don't feel guilty about making time for yourself after the baby is born. Remember that the better care you give yourself, the better care you can give your baby.

4. Accept that any mixed feelings you might have about having another child are a very real part of who you are. Do not be afraid of them, and do not try to pretend they don't exist. Ambivalence and uncertainty are a natural part of this major life transition. Talk about these feelings with someone who cares.

5. Develop a contingency plan in case PPD does recur. This may include contingencies for resuming active treatment (whatever worked for you before—e.g., therapy, medication, support group, play group), alternatives for child care, the possibility of giving up breastfeeding, and/or mobilizing family resources.

6. Give some thought to the age span between your children. We recommend waiting until your first child is three to four years old before having a second. If the spacing is too close, it puts excessive demands on the mother. Further, it is hard on your older child. If you get depressed again, a four-year-old child can handle it better than a two-year-old. It is easier to keep older children busy, it is easier to distract them, and it is easier to leave them at a friend's house.

7. Remember: no matter how prepared you are, you may still get a recurrence of PPD. You cannot "prepare" to change your biologic predisposition (except by biologic measures such as medication). But your awareness and ability to get help for yourself as soon as possible will aid your recovery.

If you have a recurrence, beginning whatever treatment was successful for you before will be most effective if it is started at the earliest sign of PPD.

*"Now that I'm feeling better, I've thought about telling people about my experience with PPD, but I'm still not sure they'll understand. Should I just try to put it all behind me?"*

Many women find that some of the shame and guilt they experienced during PPD sneaks back every once in a while after they have recovered. The stigma attached to PPD makes many women reluctant to admit they had it. However, there is evidence that women who talk about their PPD experience, especially to other women who have had similar experiences, will feel more confident and better about themselves in the long run. In fact, some women remark that the farther along they are in recovery, the more likely they are to adopt a casual attitude in their discussion of PPD, thus putting some closure on the entire episode.

*"Now that I have had PPD, can I have more children?"*

Earlier, we discussed the fact that you must consider the possibility of a recurrence of PPD if you are planning more children. With this information in hand, the question about having more children often raises painful issues.

Because deep-seated emotions, family expectations, religious values, and social norms contribute to your feelings about "ideal" family size, we recommend active discussion with your husband, your mother, other relatives who may have helped you through this crisis, and your therapist before coming to a decision. We also feel that this decision is best made when your recovery is solidly established.

Your doctor or therapist may be able to provide useful information about your decision, but because forecasting recurrences is so difficult, be sure to ask what information they considered in making a recommendation. One issue that you should consider is how seriously ill you were. For example, a woman who made a suicide attempt during an episode of PPD should be hesitant to take such a risk again, whereas in retrospect, a woman who experienced a stress syndrome may feel the risk is worth it.

You may find some surprising answers when you ask those around you how they feel about you having another baby. Your wonderful mother-in-law, who helped you tirelessly during this past crisis, may say, "Once was enough for me—I hope you don't expect me to help again." Or, she may feel that the extra effort she might have to contribute would be well worth another grandchild: "Honey, if you can get through it again, surely I can, too." Many women with PPD are excessively concerned about whether their husbands want another child, especially if they had a girl and he wanted a boy or vice versa, but find that their husbands are far more flexible than they had imagined. If you go on to have another child, and you do have a recurrence of PPD, you will feel much less guilty if others have committed their support to you in advance. Likewise, if you make the decision to limit your family size, you will also feel more comfortable about the decision if you and your husband have talked about it at length.

## Mastering PPD

Many women believe that nothing good can possibly come out of the devastation of enduring a depression after the birth of a baby. Although people may tell you that you will be stronger because of this experience, it is understandably difficult to find any positive aspects to having suffered postpartum depression.

Because the illness is such an emotional assault—a violation of what is expected to be joyful and natural—it is easy to become embittered by the experience of PPD, or to seal it over and try to forget it ever happened. Yet, by shifting your perspective, you may find some meaning in the mourning of lost hopes.

Motherhood, by definition, involves impossible expectations. Each of us longs to become the perfect mother, always to give selflessly to our children, and never to deplete our capacity to nurture those we love. But it seems that we all must wrestle this truth: the harder we aim for perfection, the less likely we are to find it.

Only when we learn that taking care of ourselves is as necessary as taking care of our families; only when we begin to accept ourselves, imperfections and all; only when we permit ourselves to face the limits of what we can do for the people we love do we achieve our fullest potential as mothers. Our children's self-esteem is linked to our own. As we learn to accept ourselves as we are, we guide our children in their journey toward loving themselves as we love them, flaws and all.

By examining the physical, hormonal, emotional, biochemical, and environmental influences in the postpartum period, we are often left with more questions than answers. Until recently, traditional theories and explanations of postpartum illnesses were ambiguous and misleading. The future of postpartum research promises to validate the struggles of many women today, by taking their needs seriously and searching for the answers that make sense. Women's issues are indeed getting more notice than in previous years. We are hopeful that old views will continue to be challenged and make way for useful new information.

Certainly, the increase of research into women's health is refreshing. But it in no way diminishes the pain of each individual woman. Women with PPD have unquestionably endured a great loss. Through experience of this loss, however, many women are able to redefine earlier expectations and, by doing so, create a new image of themselves and their families. After endless tears and fretful days, sometimes hanging in there is the best thing you can do. There is enormous power to be found in perseverance. After you succeed in waiting it out, working it through, and wondering what it's all for—you will look back. And you may see a delightfully sweet baby patiently awaiting your touch. You may see a husband who stood by you and a relationship that has been strengthened by the crisis you have surmounted together. And you may see a new you: someone who has found new dimensions to herself by overcoming this tremendous challenge.

# Recommended Reading

These are books we often recommend to our clients.

Barret, Nina. *I Wish Someone Had Told Me*. New York: Simon & Schuster, 1990.

Burns, David D. *Feeling Good*. New York: New American Library, 1981.

Davis, Valerie Raskin. *When Words Are Not Enough*. New York: Broadway Books, 1997.

———. *Great Sex for Moms*. New York: Touchstone, 2002.

———. *The Making of a Mother*. New York: Ballantine Books, 2008.

Dowling, Colette. *You Mean I Don't Have to Feel This Way?* New York: Bantam Books, 1993.

Foa, Edna, and Reid Wilson. *Stop Obsessing!* New York: Bantam Books, 1991.

Kleiman, Karen. *Dropping the Baby and Other Scary Thoughts*. New York: Routledge, 2010.

———. *The Postpartum Husband*. Bloomington, IN: xlibris, 2001.

———. *Therapy and the Postpartum Woman*. New York: Routledge, 2009.

———. *What Am I Thinking: Having a Baby After Postpartum Depression*. Bloomington, IN: xlibris, 2005.

———. *Tokens of Affection*. New York: Routledge, forthcoming.

Lerner, Harriet Goldner. *The Dance of Anger*. New York: Harper & Row, 1985.

McConnell, Patty. *A Workbook for Healing: Adult Children of Alcoholics.* San Francisco: Harper & Row, 1986.

Napthali, Sarah. *Buddhism for Mothers: A Calm Approach to Caring for Yourself and Your Children.* Australia: Allen & Unwin, 2003.

Nonacs, Ruta. *A Deeper Shade of Blue: A Woman's Guide to Recognizing and Treating Depression in Her Childbearing Years.* New York: Simon & Schuster, 2007.

Serani, Deborah. *Living with Depression: Why Biology and Biography Matter Along the Path to Hope and Healing.* New York: Rowman & Littlefield Publishers, 2011.

Shields, Brooke. *Down Came the Rain.* New York: Hyperion, 2006.

Sichel, Deborah, and Jeanne Driscoll. *Women's Moods, Women's Minds: What Every Woman Must Know About Hormones, the Brain, and Emotional Health.* New York: HarperCollins, 2000.

Tannen, Deborah. *You Just Don't Understand: Women and Men in Conversation.* New York: Ballantine, 1990.

Tolle, Ekhart. *The Power of Now.* Novato, CA: New World Library, 2004.

Twomey, Theresa. *Understanding Postpartum Psychosis.* New York: Praeger, 2009.

Viorst, Judith. *Necessary Losses.* New York: Simon & Schuster, 1986.

Weekes, Claire. *Hope and Help for Your Nerves.* New York: Bantam Books, 1969.

Weissbluth, Marc. *Healthy Sleep Habits, Happy Child.* New York: Fawcett Columbine, 1987.

Wiegartz, Pamela. *The Pregnancy and Postpartum Anxiety Workbook.* Oakland, CA: New Harbinger, 2009.

# RESOURCES

**Postpartum Support International (PSI)**

    www.postpartum.net

**Postpartum Depression Alliance of Illinois (PPD IL)**

    www.ppdil.org

**The Postpartum Stress Center, LLC**

    www.postpartumstress.com

**The Postpartum Resource Center of New York, Inc.**

    www.postpartumny.org

**Massachusetts General Hospital Center for Women's Mental Health**

    www.womensmentalhealth.org

**Postpartum Progress**

    www.postpartumprogress.com

**PostpartumMen**

    www.postpartummen.com

**The Little Angel Fund, Inc.**

    www.littleangelfund.org

**National Suicide Prevention Lifeline**

    1-800-273-TALK, 1-800-273-8255

# About the Authors

**KAREN KLEIMAN, MSW, LCSW,** is well known as an international expert on postpartum depression. In 1988, she founded The Postpartum Stress Center, LLC, a treatment and training facility for prenatal and postpartum depression and anxiety disorders where she treats individuals and couples experiencing perinatal mood and anxiety disorders. In 2009, she founded The Postpartum Stress & Family Wellness Center, LLC, in New Jersey.

In 1980, Karen received her master's in social work from the University of Illinois at Chicago and has practiced psychotherapy since that time. In addition to her clinical practice, she teaches a quarterly postgraduate training course for clinicians who have an interest in specializing in the treatment of women with postpartum depression and offers professional consultation and supervision.

Her other books include: *The Postpartum Husband: Practical Solutions for Living with Postpartum Depression; What Am I Thinking? Having a Baby After Postpartum Depression; Dropping the Baby and Other Scary Thoughts: Breaking the Cycle of Unwanted Thoughts in Motherhood* (with A. Wenzel); and *Therapy and the Postpartum Woman: Notes on Healing Postpartum Depression for Clinicians and the Women Who Seek Their Help*. Additionally, she has contributed to two parenting collections, *Parent School: Simple Lessons from the Leading Experts on Being a Mom and Dad* and *The Experts' Guide to the Baby Years*, with inserts from the perspective of a postpartum expert. She is working on her upcoming books, *Tokens of Affection: Reclaiming Your Marriage After Postpartum Depression* (with A. Wenzel) and *Cognitive Behavioral Therapy for Perinatal Distress* (with A. Wenzel).

VALERIE DAVIS (RASKIN), MD, (also known as Valerie Davis, MD) is a regional medical officer–psychiatrist with the United States Foreign Service. She was formerly an associate professor of psychiatry at the Loyola Stritch School of Medicine and chief of the psychiatry service at the Hines Veterans Administration Hospital, where she worked in the Women's Health Clinic. She has twenty-five years of experience working with mothers, including cofounding the women's psychiatry service in the Department of Psychiatry at the University of Illinois College of Medicine at Chicago. A graduate of Brown University and the University of Cincinnati College of Medicine, she completed her residency and chief residency in adult psychiatry at the University of Illinois at Chicago in 1988. Her postdoctoral research fellowship in human development at the University of Chicago concerned patterns of postpartum depression in couples. She is the mother of three young adults.

She has authored three other books: *When Words Are Not Enough: The Women's Prescription for Depression and Anxiety; Great Sex for Moms: Ten Steps to Nurturing Passion While Raising Kids;* and *The Making of a Mother: Overcoming the Nine Key Challenges, from Crib to Empty Nest.*

# INDEX